The SAC Classification in Implant Dentistry

The SAC Classification in
Implant Dentistry

The SAC Classification in Implant Dentistry

Editors:
A. Dawson, S. Chen

Authors:
A. Dawson, S. Chen,
D. Buser, L. Cordaro,
W. Martin, U. Belser

Quintessence Publishing Co, Ltd
Berlin, Chicago, London, Tokyo, Barcelona,
Beijing, Istanbul, Milan, Moscow, Mumbai,
Paris, Prague, São Paulo, Seoul, Warsaw

German National Library CIP Data

The German National Library has listed this publication in the German National Bibliography.
Detailed bibliographical data are available on the Internet at http://dnb.ddb.de.

© 2009 Quintessence Publishing Co, Ltd
Komturstraße 18, 12099 Berlin,
www.quintessenz.de

Coordination: Ä. Klebba (QPC Berlin)
Illustrations: U. Drewes (www.drewes.ch)
Graphic Concept: Wirz Corporate AG, CH-Zurich
Production: H. Rohde (QPC Berlin)
Printing: Bosch-Druck GmbH
                  (www.bosch-druck.de)

Printed in Germany
ISBN: 978-1-85097-188-7

Acknowledgement

The authors wish to express their sincere thanks to Ms. Ute Drewes for the artwork and illustrations in this textbook and to Ms. Jeannie Wurz for her excellent assistance during the editing process. We would also like to thank Straumann Holding AG, our corporate partner, for their unwavering and ongoing support of the activities and publications of the ITI.

Foreword

The rapid development of clinical techniques and biomaterials in implant dentistry has led to an expansion in the clinical indications for this modality of treatment. Implant dentistry now forms an integral part of everyday dental practice. However, education in implant dentistry for most dentists occurs after graduation with little emphasis on the identification of treatment complexity and risks. Since 2003, the International Team for Implantology (ITI) has recommended the SAC Classification to categorize treatment procedures into three levels of difficulty - *Straightforward*, *Advanced* and *Complex*.

In March 2007, the ITI organized a conference involving a multi-disciplinary group of 28 clinicians who met in Mallorca, Spain to standardize the application of the SAC Classification. The ITI is proud to be able to publish the proceedings of the conference in this volume.

The aim of the ITI is to promote and disseminate knowledge in all aspects of implant dentistry and related tissue regeneration. Together with the ITI Treatment Guide series, this book furthers the desire of the ITI to support the development of practical tools for clinicians and educators in dental implantology. The ITI recommends this book to all professionals in this field.

Dieter Weingart
ITI President

Stephen Chen
Chairman,
ITI Education Committee

Editors and Authors

Editors/Authors

Anthony Dawson, MDS
   Suite 7, 12 Napier Close
   Deakin, ACT, 2600, Australia
   E-mail: tony@canberraprosthodontics.com.au

Stephen Chen, MDSc, PhD
   The University of Melbourne
   School of Dental Science
   720 Swanston Street
   Melbourne, VIC 3010, Australia
   E-Mail: schen@balwynperio.com.au

Authors

Daniel Buser, DMD, Professor
   University of Berne
   Department of Oral Surgery and Stomatology
   School of Dental Medicine
   Freiburgstrasse 7, 3010 Bern, Switzerland
   E-Mail: daniel.buser@zmk.unibe.ch

Luca Cordaro MD, DDS, PhD
   Eastman Dental Hospital, Roma
   Head: Department of Periodontics and
   Prosthodontics
   Via Guido D' Arezzo 2, Roma 00198, Italy
   E-mail: lucacordaro@usa.net

William C. Martin, DMD, MS
   University of Florida, College of Dentistry
   Clinical Associate Professor,
   Center for Implant Dentistry
   Department of Oral and Maxillofacial Surgery
   1600 W Archer Road, D7-6, Gainesville, FL 32610, USA
   E-Mail: wmartin@dental.ufl.edu

Urs C. Belser, DMD, Professor
   University of Geneva
   Department of Prosthodontics
   School of Dental Medicine
   Rue Barthélemy-Menn 19, 1211 Genève 4, Switzerland
   E-Mail: urs.belser@medecine.unige.ch

Contributors

Contributors

Arne F. Boeckler
Martin-Luther-University Halle-Wittenberg
Associate Professor
Department of Prosthodontics
Grosse Steinstrasse 19, 06108 Halle (Saale)
Germany
E-Mail: arne.boeckler@medizin.uni-halle.de

Anthony J. Dickinson, BDSc, MSD
1564 Malvern Road
Glen Iris, VIC 3146, Australia
E-Mail: ajd1@iprimus.com.au

Christopher Evans, BDSc Hons (Qld), MDSc (Melb)
75 Asling St., Brighton
Melbourne, VIC 3186, Australia
E-Mail: cdjevans@mac.com

Hidekazu Hayashi, DDS, PhD
Family Dental Clinic
2 Saki-cho Nara, Nara 630-8003, Japan
E-Mail: Hide1@nike.eonet.ne.jp

Frank Higginbottom, DDS
3600 Gaston Avenue, Suite 1107
Dallas, TX 75246, USA
E-Mail: bottom@dallasesthetics.com

Dean Morton, BDS, MS
University of Louisville, School of Dentistry
Professor and Assistant Dean
Department of Diagnostic Sciences, Prosthodontics
and Restorative Dentistry
501 S. Preston, Louisville, KY 40292, USA
E-Mail: dean.morton@louisville.edu

Zahra Rashid, BSc, DDS, MS, FRCD (C), FCDS (BC)
1466 West Hastings Street
Vancouver, BC, V6G 3J6, Canada
E-Mail: zrashid@shaw.ca

James Ruskin, DMD, MD
University of Florida, College of Dentistry
Professor and Director, Center for Implant Dentistry
Department of Oral And Maxillofacial Surgery
1600 W Archer Road, D7-6, Gainesville, FL 32610, USA
E-Mail: jruskin@dental.ufl.edu

Thomas G. Wilson Jr, DDS, PA
Periodontics and Dental Implants
5465 Blair Road, Suite 200
Dallas, TX 75231, USA
E-Mail: tom@tgwperio.com

Table of Contents

1 An Introduction to the SAC Classification

A. Dawson, S. Chen, D. Buser

1.1   Introduction

Over the past 15 years, implant dentistry has progressed to become the standard of care for the rehabilitation of fully and partially edentulous patients. Clinical and technological advances have led to an expansion of the indications for implant therapy, providing increased opportunities for dental practitioners to become involved in the delivery of care. Along with these advances there has been an increase in the complexity of treatment being recommended to patients. This has increased the need for clinicians in the field of implant dentistry to be able to provide surgical and restorative therapy at an appropriate level of care.

It has long been recognized that clinical situations present with different levels of difficulty, and with different degrees of risk for esthetic, restorative and surgical complications. To date, there is no widely accepted classification system in implant dentistry aimed at defining the level of treatment complexity and the potential for complica-

tions. To assist clinicians in evaluating the degree of difficulty of individual cases, the International Team for Implantology (ITI) organized a Consensus Conference in Palma de Mallorca, Spain, from March 13th to 15th, 2007. The aim of the conference was to provide guidelines for various types of restorative and surgical cases based on a system referred to as the *Straightforward*, *Advanced* and *Complex* classification system (SAC).

These guidelines will provide clinicians with a reference for selecting appropriate cases and planning implant therapy. As well, this book will serve as a useful tool for academics wishing to design implant training programs with incremental levels of difficulty.

1.2 List of Consensus Conference Participants

This text documents the proceedings of a SAC Consensus Conference held by the International Team for Implantology (ITI) in Palma de Mallorca, Spain, over the period March 13th to 15th, 2007. The following individuals contributed to the consensus statements of this conference and the content of this publication:

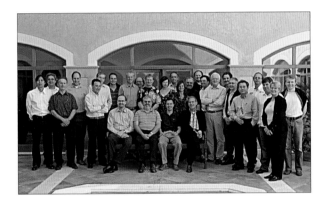

Urs Belser	Switzerland	Alessandro Januário	Brazil
Daniele Botticelli	Italy	Simon Jensen	Denmark
Daniel Buser	Switzerland	Hideaki Katsuyama	Japan
Stephen Chen	Australia	Christian Krenkel	Austria
Luca Cordaro	Italy	Richard Leesungbok	South Korea
Anthony Dawson	Australia	Will Martin	USA
Anthony Dickinson	Australia	Lisa Heitz-Mayfield	Australia
Javier G. Fabrega	Spain	Dean Morton	USA
Andreas Feloutzis	Greece	Helena Rebelo	Portugal
Kerstin Fischer	Sweden	Paul Rousseau	France
Christoph Hämmerle	Switzerland	Bruno Schmid	Switzerland
Timothy Head	Canada	Hendrik Terheyden	Germany
Frank Higginbottom	USA	Adrian Watkinson	UK
Haldun Iplikcioglu	Turkey	Daniel Wismeijer	Netherlands

1.3 Introduction to the SAC Classification

The SAC Classification is an assessment of the potential difficulty and risk of a case, and serves as a guide for clinicians in both case selection and treatment planning. Classifications of *Straightforward* (low difficulty and low risk), *Advanced* (moderate difficulty and moderate risk), and *Complex* (high difficulty and high risk) may be assigned to a case for both restorative and surgical aspects. The knowledge, skill and experience of individual clinicians, however, introduces subjectivity by influencing their perception of what a specific case may be classified as. The aim of this book is to bring objectivity to this process with respect to the "standard" presentation of clinical cases. It should be recognized, however, that the classification of individual cases may be altered as a consequence of modifying factors. These factors will be outlined in later chapters of this book.

The first SAC Classification was described by Sailer and Pajarola in an atlas of oral surgery (Sailer and Pajarola 1999). The authors described in detail various clinical situations for procedures in oral surgery, such as the removal of third molars, and proposed the classification S = *Simple*, A = *Advanced*, and C = *Complex*. The SAC Classification was then adopted in 1999 by the Swiss Society of Oral Implantology (SSOI) during a one-week congress on quality guidelines in dentistry. The working group of the SSOI developed this SAC Classification from a surgical and prosthetic point of view for various clinical situations in implant dentistry. This SAC Classification was then adopted by the International Team for Implantology in 2003 during the ITI Consensus Conference in Gstaad, Switzerland. The surgical SAC Classification was presented in the proceedings of this conference (Buser et al. 2004). The ITI Education Core Group decided in 2006 to slightly modify the original classification by changing the term *Simple* to *Straightforward*.

The following chapter provides a review of the SAC Classification, its applications and its determinants. Criteria for categorization of case types were established, and normative classifications (see the following chapter for definitions) for individual case types were assigned. Subsequent chapters will detail the application of the SAC Classification in the surgical and restorative fields of implant dentistry. The effects of modifying factors and complications on the normative classification of cases will also be presented and discussed.

Although it is primarily designed as a guide for identification of the level of difficulty of individual cases, the SAC Classification may also be used as a tool for risk identification and patient management. Patients may be prepared for treatment by being given information on expected limitations, complications and outcomes based on the SAC Classification. This in turn would allow patients to form realistic expectations of the potential outcome of therapy. Consequently, the SAC Classification has a number of potential audiences and uses. For novice implant clinicians, the SAC Classification provides a case selection and treatment planning tool which can help them develop their experience in implant dentistry in a responsible and incremental manner. More experienced clinicians may find somewhat less use in these areas, but might find this a useful framework for planning implant treatments and for identifying, and thus potentially controlling, risk.

The SAC Classification may also be applied throughout the treatment process. A normative classification, based on the site and type of clinical presentation, may be altered by patient-specific factors. The assigned classification may be further modified during the active treatment phases, if required.

2 The Determinants of the SAC Classification

A. Dawson, S. Chen

2.1 Definitions

Table 1. Classification of the Timing of Implant Placement following Tooth Extraction (Chen and Buser 2008).

Classification	Descriptive Terminology	Period after Tooth Extraction	Desired Clinical Situation at Implant Placement
Type 1	Immediate placement	Immediately following extraction	Post-extraction site with no healing of bone or soft tissues
Type 2	Early placement with soft-tissue healing	Typically 4 to 8 weeks	Post-extraction site with healed soft tissue but without significant bone healing
Type 3	Early placement with partial bone healing	Typically 12 to 16 weeks	Post-extraction site with healed soft tissues and with significant bone healing
Type 4	Late placement	Typically 6 months or longer	Fully healed post-extraction site

Process: The implant dentistry "process" is defined as the full range of issues pertaining to assessment, planning, management of treatment, and subsequent maintenance of the implant and prosthetic reconstruction; it does not merely refer to the clinical treatment procedures that are involved.

Normative: In this context, "normative" relates to the classification that conforms to the norm, or standard, for a given clinical situation in implant dentistry. The normative classification relates to the most likely representation of the classification of a case. The normative classification may alter as a result of modifying factors and/or complications.

Timing of implant placement: A number of different classifications have been used to describe the timing of implant placement after tooth extraction. In this book, the classification detailed by Chen and Buser (2008), which is a modification of the classification proposed by Hämmerle et al. (2004), will be used. This classification is summarized in Table 1.

Implant loading protocol: In discussions relating to the systems for loading implants after implant placement, the definitions used by Cochran et al. (2004) will be used. These are summarized in Table 2.

Table 2. Definitions of Loading Protocols (Cochran et al. 2004).

Loading Protocol	Definition
Immediate restoration	A restoration is inserted within 48 hours of implant placement, but not in occlusion with the opposing dentition
Immediate loading	A restoration is placed in occlusion with the opposing dentition within 48 hours of implant placement
Conventional loading	The prosthesis is attached after a healing period of 3 to 6 months
Early loading	A restoration in contact with the opposing dentition is placed at least 48 hours after implant placement but not later than 3 months afterwards
Delayed Loading	The prosthesis is attached in a procedure that takes place some time later than the conventional healing period of 3 to 6 months

2.2 Assumptions

This classification assumes that appropriate training, preparation and care are devoted to the planning and implementation of treatment plans. No classification can adequately address cases or outcomes that deviate significantly from the norm. In addition, it is assumed that clinicians will be practicing within the bounds of their clinical competence and abilities. Thus, within each classification, the following general and specific assumptions are implied:

General:

- Treatment will be provided in an appropriately equipped operatory with an appropriate aseptic technique.
- Adequate clinical and laboratory support is available.
- Recommended protocols are followed.

Patients:

- Patients' medical conditions are not compromised or are appropriately addressed.
- Patients have realistic expectations with respect to the outcomes of their treatment.

Specific:

- The type, dimensions and number of implants to be placed are appropriate for the site.
- The implants are correctly positioned and adequately spaced.
- Restorative materials that are used are appropriate to the task.

2.3   Determinants of Classification

The normative classification for a given type of case will be determined based on the criteria outlined below.

General determinants of classification include:

2.3.1   Esthetic vs. Non-Esthetic Sites

The extent to which esthetic issues affect the process will be a general determinant. Cases in non-esthetic sites will have little or no esthetic risk, thus removing one potentially confounding factor. *Straightforward* cases must not, by definition, include any esthetic risk, and any case in the esthetic zone must be classified as either *Advanced* or *Complex*. In this context, an esthetic site is one in which the mucosal margins of teeth or tooth replacements will be visible upon full smile, or an area of esthetic importance to the patient (Belser et al. 2004).

2.3.2   Complexity of the Process

The level of complexity of an implant surgical or restorative treatment may be assessed by considering the number of steps involved in the procedure, and the number of areas in which an appropriate outcome must be achieved. As a general principle, the level of complexity rises with an increase in the number of steps involved and the number of objectives that must be achieved to attain a satisfactory result.

For example, a single-tooth replacement in a non-esthetic site may require limited planning. Surgery may involve an uncomplicated two-step process involving tooth extraction and subsequent implant placement some weeks later. The restorative phase of treatment may also involve an uncomplicated procedure. This case would, therefore, have a normative classification of *Straightforward* for both the surgical and restorative treatments. In contrast, a single-tooth restoration in an esthetic site will require more detailed assessment and planning, may involve more surgical and restorative steps, and must achieve somewhat more exacting outcomes. This process would have a normative classification of at least *Advanced*. While seemingly similar in application, these two examples demonstrate the increased complexity that attends cases in esthetically challenging sites.

Assessment of the complexity of a process can also be based on whether the outcome (and steps involved) can be predicted with some clarity. If they can, then classifications of *Straightforward* or *Advanced* may be appropriate (depending on other issues under consideration). In *Complex* cases the outcome is likely to be dependent on the success of intermediate procedures. This may require variations in the treatment plan and consideration of the associated contingencies. For example, if sinus grafting is necessary to place implants, the outcome of the procedure will, to a greater or lesser degree, affect the number, size and placement of implants, which in turn will affect the design of the final prosthesis. Thus, in the planning phase it is not possible to clearly envision the final outcome, leading to a classification of *Complex*.

2.3.3   Risks of Complications

No procedure is totally without risk of a mishap that may complicate the treatment or affect the long-term success and stability of the result. The SAC Classification can be used to identify and quantify these risks, thus allowing some contingency planning to be undertaken to control risk and minimize undesirable outcomes. In this sense, the SAC Classification can serve as a valuable risk management tool for dental practitioners.

Complications may lead to one or more of the following outcomes:

- The complication makes the surgical and/or restorative treatment more difficult, but does not have any effect on the outcome;
- The complication results in a sub-optimal outcome which does not reduce the survival of the resulting restoration, but the result falls short of accepted ideals in one or more areas;
- The complication compromises the outcome to the extent that long-term success or stability of the final restoration is diminished (Figure 1); or
- The complication results in failure of the procedure.

Where risks are identified during the assessment and planning phases of the treatment process, measures can be initiated and included in the treatment plan to minimize the undesirable outcomes of potentially negative events. Patients can be counseled regarding these risks and warned of the potential down-side. Expectations can be controlled and patients prepared for sub-optimal outcomes should they arise.

What are areas of potential risk? The following list indicates broad areas that may influence the degree of difficulty of a clinical process, and thus the attendant SAC Classification:

- Biological factors:
  - Hard and soft tissue volume
  - Amount of keratinized mucosa
  - Presence of infection
  - Occlusal factors (e.g., occlusal parafunction)
- Technical factors:
  - Restoration design
  - Laboratory issues
- Esthetic factors:
  - Esthetic Risk Assessment (Martin et al. 2007)
  - The need to replace missing soft tissue volume in an esthetic site
- Patient factors:
  - Esthetic needs or expectations exceed what can reasonably be achieved
  - Willingness of patients to commit to their role in the treatment plan
  - Compliance
- Process factors:
  - Issues that relate to the number of steps involved in the process, or the complexity of those steps
  - Factors that may impact on the coordination or scheduling of treatment processes. For example, immediate loading treatments tend to be more demanding with respect to scheduling and logistic considerations.

These issues will be considered in more detail later in this text. However, during the case assessment and selection phase of management, the potential for these types of complications must be considered. It is this "potential" which contributes to the normative SAC Classification.

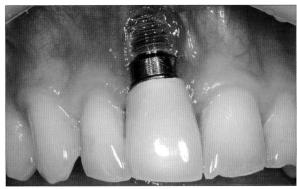

Figure 1.   Facial view of an implant in the upper right central incisor site showing mucosal recession and loss of bone support on the facial aspect. The implant is over-sized and was placed in a facial malposition in the extraction socket. This complication has adversely affected esthetic success and has compromised the long-term survival of the implant.

3 <u>Modifying Factors</u>

3.1 General Modifiers

S. Chen, A. Dawson

Normative classifications refer only to standard presentations of a case type. The following factors may modify these classifications, generally through increasing the difficulty of a treatment process:

3.1.1 Clinical Competence and Experience

While it is assumed that clinicians will undertake implant therapy that does not exceed their clinical abilities, it should be noted that the normative SAC Classification for a case type is independent of the clinicians' skill and competence. Thus, a *Straightforward* case will represent an uncomplicated procedure for both the novice and experienced clinician. On the other hand, a *Complex* case will be difficult to manage for the novice and experienced clinician alike. In this regard, the difference between the two is that the experienced clinician possesses the skill, competence and knowledge to manage the complex case and to deal with complications should they arise. In contrast, the novice clinician lacks the necessary skill and experience and would be best advised to refer such a case to someone with greater expertise.

3.1.2 Compromised Patient Health

Treatment of patients with compromised health is often more difficult in execution as well as more prone to complications (Table 1). For example, we know that smokers (Strietzel et al. 2007) and patients with uncontrolled diabetes mellitus (Moy et al. 2005, Ferreira et al. 2006) are more likely to have post-operative complications and im-

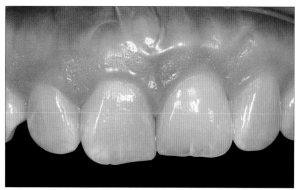

Figure 1. Three years after implant placement, there is a discrepancy in the level of the incisal edges of the implant in the 21 site and the adjacent central incisor due to dento-facial growth.

plant failure and are regarded as at high risk for implant therapy. Other conditions can also have an impact in these areas, and must be assessed during the work-up for each case. These factors may be controlled to allow progression of the treatment, but the treatment process generally requires variations from standard treatment protocols.

Table 1. General Risk Factors in Candidates for Implant Therapy (Buser et al. 2004).

Risk Factor	Remarks
Medical	• Severe bone disease causing impaired bone healing • Immunological disease • Medication with steroids • Uncontrolled diabetes mellitus • Irradiated bone • Others
Periodontal	• Active periodontal disease • History of refractive periodontitis • Genetic predisposition
Oral Hygiene/Compliance	• Home care measured by gingival indices • Personality, intellectual aspects
Occlusion	• Bruxism

3.1.3 Growth Considerations

Implants placed into the jaws of growing individuals represent a significant modifying factor. Experimental studies (Thilander et al. 1992) and clinical case reports in growing patients (Oesterle et al. 1993, Johansson et al. 1994, Westwood and Duncan 1996) have shown that implants act in a similar manner to ankylosed teeth by retarding the growth of the alveolar process in the immediate vicinity of the implant. The net effect is a relative infraocclusion and/or palatoversion of the implant (Figure 1). The clinical presentations of this are not only associated with esthetic issues (mismatch of incisal edges and gingival margins between the implant restoration and the contralateral tooth) but also with functional issues where restorations move into infraocclusion.

For these reasons, placement of implants should be postponed in young individuals until craniofacial/skeletal growth is complete (Koch et al. 1996). However, the growth period varies widely in children, and chronological age alone should not be used as a criterion. It has been recommended that a combination of methods be used to determine growth cessation, including serial cephalometric tracings, tooth eruption patterns within the arch (e.g., eruption of the second molar), evaluation of bodily growth in length, and evaluation of hand/wrist radiographs (Op Heij et al. 2003). It should be noted that individuals with a short or long face type may demonstrate further eruption of teeth adjacent to implants after the age of 20 years, posing a risk to esthetic and functional outcomes (Op Heij et al. 2006).

There is evidence that craniofacial growth may never cease completely, but may slowly continue throughout life (Behrents 1985). Over time, adaptive changes in tooth position may affect esthetics and function, requiring modification to or replacement of the implant-supported prostheses in mature adults (Oesterle and Cronin 2000).

3.1.4 Iatrogenic Factors

Sub-optimal planning, as well as less-than-desirable outcomes in preceding treatment procedures, will often increase the difficulty of implant treatment phases. For example, implant placement into an upper lateral incisor site is more difficult when orthodontic treatment has failed to make sufficient space between the roots of adjacent teeth. Sub-optimal three-dimensional implant placement will also complicate the restorative process (Buser et al. 2004), and likely alter the classification for that particular presentation (Figures 2 to 7).

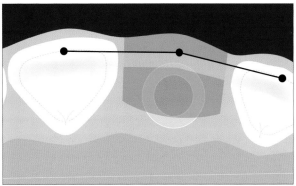

Figure 2.   Schematic drawing of the orofacial comfort and danger zones.

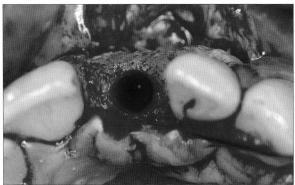

Figure 3.   Occlusal view following implant bed preparation with a proper orofacial implant position and an intact facial bone wall.

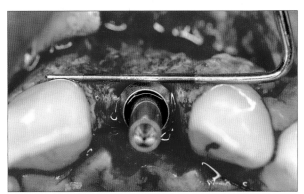

Figure 4.   Periodontal probe visualizing the correct position of the implant shoulder in orofacial direction.

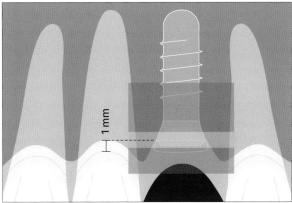

Figure 5.   Comfort and danger zones in the coronoapical dimension.

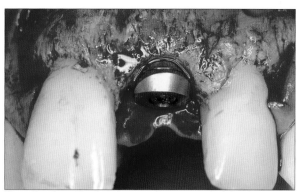

Figure 6.   Correct implant placement in a coronoapical direction.

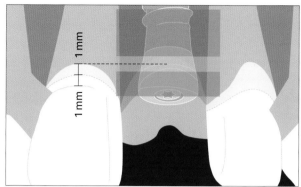

Figure 7.   Schematic drawing illustrating the comfort and danger zones in the coronoapical dimension.

3.2 Esthetic Modifiers

S. Chen, A. Dawson

Esthetic issues apply where the implant restoration, and the surrounding mucosal margin, will be visible during normal functional activity or when the patient smiles. Consequently, not all implant treatments will have associated esthetic risk. This series of modifiers has been discussed in detail in *"The ITI Treatment Guide, Volume 1: Implant Therapy in the Esthetic Zone – Single Tooth Replacements"* (Martin et al. 2007).

Table 1 lists the factors that determine esthetic risk. This Esthetic Risk Assessment (ERA) can be used to determine the risk of a negative esthetic outcome for a particular treatment, thus assisting the clinician in determining the SAC Classification of the case. It should be noted that, by definition, a case for which there is some esthetic risk (i.e.

the restoration margin is visible) would have a classification of at least *Advanced*.

The factors listed in the ERA all affect the volume and health of the hard and soft tissues that surround implant restorations, and how these are likely to influence esthetic outcomes. An implant restoration in an esthetically demanding site can be compared to a painting in an art gallery. The surrounding soft tissues, and the bone that supports them, are analogous to the frame surrounding the painting. The overall esthetic effect of this piece of art will be enhanced by a good frame, but can be significantly degraded by a poor one. It is the same with an implant restoration.

Table 1. Esthetic Risk Assessment (ERA).

Esthetic Risk Factor	Level of Risk		
	Low	Moderate	High
Medical status	Healthy, co-operative patient with an intact immune system.		Reduced immune system
Smoking habit	Non-smoker	Light smoker (< 10 cigs/day)	Heavy smoker (> 10 cigs/day)
Patient's esthetic expectations	Low	Medium	High
Lip line	Low	Medium	High
Gingival biotype	Low scalloped, thick	Medium scalloped, medium thick	High scalloped, thin
Shape of tooth crowns	Rectangular		Triangular
Infection at implant site	None	Chronic	Acute
Bone level at adjacent teeth	≤ 5 mm to contact point	5.5 to 6.5 mm to contact point	≥ 7 mm to contact point
Restorative status of neighboring teeth	Virgin		Restored
Width of edentulous span	1 tooth (≥ 7 mm)	1 tooth (≤ 7mm)	2 teeth or more
Soft tissue anatomy	Intact soft tissue		Soft tissue defects
Bone anatomy of alveolar crest	Alveolar crest without bone deficiency	Horizontal bone deficiency	Vertical bone deficiency

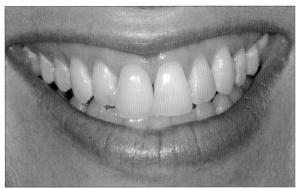

Figure 1. *Facial view of a patient with a high smile line. The blunting of the papilla between the implant in the 21 site and the adjacent central incisor is visible when the patient smiles.*

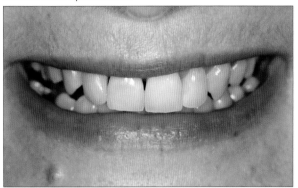

Figure 2. *Facial view of a patient with a low smile line. Although there has been loss of the papilla between the implant in the 21 site and the adjacent central incisor, this is not readily seen when the patient smiles.*

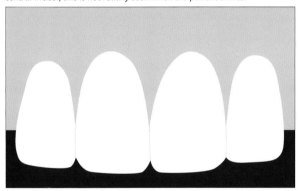

Figure 3. *Diagrammatic representation of a thin biotype. Note triangular tooth forms and high, scalloped gingival margins.*

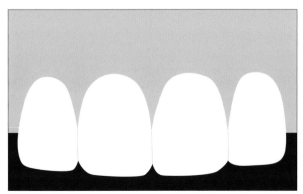

Figure 4. *Diagrammatic representation of a thick biotype. Note the more rectangular tooth forms and lower, less scalloped gingival margins.*

3.2.1   Health Status

The impact of medical issues such as health status and smoking relates primarily to the predictability of the healing process. These issues have been discussed previously.

3.2.2   Esthetic Expectations

Patients' expectations with regard to the esthetic outcome also represent a significant issue in planning esthetic cases. Patients with unrealistic demands or those whose esthetic needs are very high, may be difficult to treat as the esthetic outcome of an implant treatment may not be able to meet these expectations or needs. Patients should be fully advised as to how limitations imposed by the other factors in the ERA are likely to influence their individual outcomes, and this information must be communicated very early in the assessment and planning process. Additionally, treatment modalities other than implants should be considered if these might provide more satisfactory or predictable outcomes.

3.2.3   Smile Line

The level to which the planned implant restoration and its surrounding mucosal tissue is exposed during function and smiling is a major factor defining whether the site is considered esthetic or non-esthetic. If the peri-implant mucosal margin is not visible during function or smiling, the site would normally be considered as having little or no esthetic risk. Greater exposure of this area is associated with increasing esthetic risk (Figures 1 and 2).

3.2.4   Gingival Biotype

The soft tissue biotype may influence the esthetic outcome of implant restorations (Kois 2001). At natural teeth, the gingiva of the thin biotype is associated with highly scalloped gingival margins and more triangular tooth crowns (Figure 3), whereas for thick biotypes the gingival margins are less scalloped and the tooth crowns are more rectangular in shape (Figure 4) (Olsson et al. 1993). In addition, the zone of keratinized gingiva is wider in thick biotypes than in thin biotypes (Müller and Eger 1997).

At single tooth implants, the dimensions of the facial supra-crestal soft tissues are greater for thick tissue biotypes compared to thin tissue biotypes (Kan et al. 2003). Thin biotypes seem to be more often associated with soft tissue recession around implant restorations than thick biotypes (Evans and Chen 2008), and it can be more difficult to develop optimal soft tissue transition zones. Thicker biotypes, which are less common, appear to be more forgiving and more easily controlled. Thus the transition from thick biotype to thin biotype is associated with an increasing esthetic risk (Martin et al. 2007).

3.2.5 Volume of Surrounding Soft Tissues

Many of the factors in the ERA relate to the volume of the mucosal tissues, and supporting bone in the implant site. Their influence on implant placement and restoration in a manner that will allow the development of esthetic symmetry and harmony with surrounding teeth and soft tissues is of critical concern. Issues that might compromise this tissue volume, such as crestal bone resorption and mucosal recession, will increase the esthetic risk and the level of treatment difficulty.

Bony support for peri-implant soft tissues is critical when esthetic risk is present (Belser et al. 1998, Buser and von Arx 2000). One area where this issue has a great impact is in the support for papillae between teeth and implants (Choquet et al. 2001), or between implants (Tarnow et al. 2000, Tarnow et al. 2003). In a single-tooth case with intact papillae supported by the proximal bone crests on adjacent teeth, it is likely that the papillae can be maintained through proper implant selection and good surgical technique, thus leading to low esthetic risk. However, where bony support for the papilla is reduced by periodontal disease, deep subgingival restoration margins, or active infection, the risk of sub-optimal outcomes is much higher. This issue can also arise when the mesio-distal space for implant placement is reduced, allowing crestal remodeling to compromise this supporting bone. Longer spans, involving the replacement of multiple missing teeth, can be very difficult in terms of developing the "natural" appearance of papillae between the prosthetic teeth (Buser et al. 2004), and the use of prosthetic soft-tissue replacements may be necessary.

3.3 Surgical Modifying Factors

S. Chen, D. Buser, L. Cordaro

Table 1 outlines the modifying factors that should be considered in assessment of a potential implant site for surgical management.

3.3.1 Bone Volume

A basic requirement for implant therapy is bone volume that is sufficient to support an implant of adequate length (Buser et al. 2000). Following tooth extraction, resorptive changes result in varying patterns and degrees of bone resorption (Figures 1a and 1b), leading to reduced horizontal and vertical bone dimensions (Schropp et al. 2003). This in turn may necessitate bone augmentation procedures either prior to or at the time of implant placement. The need for adjunctive bone augmentation procedures increases the difficulty of surgical treatment.

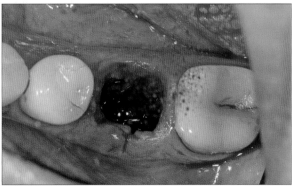

Figure 1a.   Occlusal view of a 36 extraction site immediately after removal of the tooth.

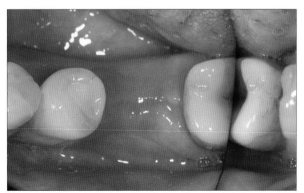

Figure 1b.   Twelve weeks later, the soft tissues have healed. There has been marked resorption on the facial aspect of the ridge.

With horizontal deficiencies, a simultaneous bone augmentation procedure may be carried out when the anticipated peri-implant defect presents with at least two bone walls (see Chapter 4 for further details). Simultaneous horizontal augmentation procedures are regarded as moderately difficult to perform, requiring skill and experience in the use of barrier membranes and/or bone grafts and bone substitutes. If the defect is anticipated to be a one-wall defect, a staged approach is recommended. Procedures associated with these types of defects – such as lateral bone augmentation with combinations of block and particulate grafts and/or space-maintaining or membrane-tenting procedures – have a high degree of difficulty and require skill and experience. There is a commensurate increase in the risk of surgical and post-operative complications.

With vertical deficiencies, small crestal bone deficiencies may be managed without augmentation; however, the implant shoulder may be deeply positioned in relation to the mucosal margin. This increases the difficulty of subsequent restorative procedures and may complicate long-term maintenance of peri-implant tissue health. If the presence of anatomical structures reduces the height of bone in the apical dimension, implants with shorter lengths than is standard for a given system may be considered. However, the long-term survival of these implants is not well documented and may be reduced. At sites with reduced bone height, the proximity to anatomic structures increases the risk of surgical complications. For these reasons, sites with vertical bone deficiencies should be regarded as having a moderate degree of difficulty for surgical management.

At sites with significant crestal or apical vertical deficiencies, techniques for vertical bone augmentation may include sinus and nasal floor grafts, vertical crestal augmentation using barrier membranes and/or bone grafts or bone substitutes, and distraction osteogenesis. These procedures have a high degree of difficulty and an increased risk of surgical complications. Clinicians require a high level of clinical skill and experience to carry out these procedures successfully.

Table 1. Surgical Modifying Factors.

Site Factors	Risk or Degree of Difficulty		
	Low	Moderate	High
Bone Volume			
Horizontal	Adequate	Deficient, but allowing simultaneous augmentation	Deficient, requiring prior augmentation
Vertical	Adequate	Small deficiency crestally, requiring slightly deeper corono-apical implant position. Small deficiency apically due to proximity to anatomical structures, requiring shorter than standard implant lengths.	Deficient, requiring prior augmentation
Anatomic Risk			
Proximity to vital anatomic structures	Minimal risk of involvement	Moderate risk of involvement	High risk of involvement
Esthetic Risk			
Esthetic zone	No		Yes
Biotype	Thick		Thin
Thickness of facial bone wall	sufficient ≥ 1 mm		insufficient < 1 mm
Complexity			
Number of prior or simultaneous procedures	Implant placement without adjunctive procedures	Implant placement with simultaneous procedures	Implant placement with staged procedures
Complications			
Risk of surgical complications	Minimal	Moderate	High
Consequences of complications	No adverse effect	Suboptimal outcome	Severely compromised outcome

3.3.2 Anatomic Risk

Implant surgery carries a risk of involvement of nearby anatomic structures such as adjacent roots, neurovascular structures, the maxillary sinus and nasal cavity, and the possibility of perforation of the cortical bone. Careful clinical and radiographic preoperative assessment of the site is required to determine the degree of risk of involvement of these structures. If bone or soft tissue is to be harvested for grafting, the anatomic risk at the donor site must also be considered. Depending upon the clinical situation, the risk may range from low to high.

3.3.3 Esthetic Risk

The assessment of esthetic risk has been outlined in section 3.2. From a surgical perspective, tissue biotype is an important determinant of risk. Compared to sites with thick tissue, sites with thin tissue are at greater risk of recession of the marginal mucosa (Evans and Chen 2008), and may frequently require adjunctive hard and soft tissue augmentation procedures to prevent this from occurring. This increases the difficulty of treatment, and requires that clinicians possess a high level of clinical skill and experience to complete these procedures successfully. Sites with thin tissues in esthetically important areas are very difficult to manage, with an elevated risk of esthetic complications.

The facial bone wall supports the mucosa on the facial aspect of the implant. If the facial bone wall is thin (< 1 mm) following installation of the implant, there is an increased risk of horizontal and vertical marginal bone resorption and exposure of the implant surface (Block and Kent 1990). This in turn increases the likelihood of marginal tissue recession. Adjunctive hard and soft tissue augmentation procedures are frequently performed to minimize the risk of marginal bone resorption and mucosal recession. Due to the higher esthetic risk, sites with thin facial bone walls have a high degree of difficulty.

3.3.4 Complexity

Implant sites that may be managed without adjunctive hard or soft tissue augmentation procedures are regarded as having a low level of difficulty. Sites that require adjunctive augmentation procedures have a moderate or high level of difficulty, depending upon the complexity and number of steps involved, and whether a simultaneous or staged approach is indicated.

3.3.5 Complications

A wide variety of surgical and augmentation techniques are available to clinicians who place implants. Clinicians must have a sound understanding of the advantages, disadvantages and clinical evidence supporting the efficacy of techniques they recommend to patients.

The risk of a complication is inherent in any surgical technique, and is influenced by a number of factors, including the complexity of the procedure, proximity to anatomic structures, esthetic factors, and the skill and experience of the clinician undertaking the treatment. The risk of complication can range from low to high, and must be assessed for each case and for the technique(s) selected.

A further consideration is the consequence of a complication. If a complication can be managed without any adverse effect on the implant or restoration, then the complication may be regarded as low risk. If the complication results in adverse bone and/or soft tissue outcomes, the risk of long-term consequences may be moderate to high (Figure 2), depending upon the nature of the complication.

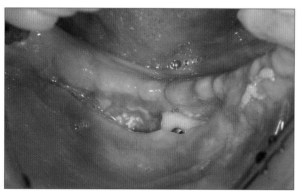

Figure 2. Clinical view of a wound dehiscence in a lower posterior site that has exposed a bone graft that was placed for lateral augmentation of the ridge.

3.4 Restorative Modifiers

A. Dawson, W. Martin

Table 1 shows details of the restorative issues and risks that might influence the SAC Classification of an individual case.

Table 1. Restorative Modifying Factors.

		Degree of Difficulty		
Issue	**Notes**	**Low**	**Moderate**	**High**
Oral Environment				
General oral health		No active disease		Active disease
Condition of adjacent teeth		Restored teeth		Virgin teeth
Reason for tooth loss		Caries/Trauma		Periodontal disease or occlusal parafunction
Restorative Volume				
Inter-arch distance	Refers to the distance from the proposed implant restorative margin to the opposing occlusion	Adequate for planned restoration	Restricted space, but can be managed	Adjunctive therapy will be necessary to gain sufficient space for the planned restoration
Mesio-distal space	The arch length available to fit tooth replacements	Sufficient to fit replacements for missing teeth	Some reduction in size or number of teeth will be necessary	Adjunctive therapy will be needed to achieve a satisfactory result
Span of restoration		Single tooth	Extended edentulous space	Full arch
Volume and characteristics of the edentulous saddle	Refers to whether there is sufficient tissue volume to support the final restoration, or some prosthetic replacement of soft tissues will be necessary.	No prosthetic soft-tissue replacement will be necessary		Prosthetic replacement of soft tissue will be needed for esthetics or phonetics

Table 1. Restorative Modifying Factors (contd.).

Issue	Notes	Degree of Difficulty		
		Low	**Moderate**	**High**
Occlusion				
Occlusal scheme		Anterior guidance		No guidance
Involvement in occlusion	The degree to which the implant prosthesis is involved in the patient's occlusal scheme	Minimal involvement		Implant restoration is involved in guidance
Occlusal parafunction	Risk of complication to the restoration, but not to implant survival	Absent		Present
Provisional Restorations				
During implant healing		None required	Removable	Fixed
Implant-supported provisionals needed	Provisional restorations will be needed to develop esthetics and soft tissue transition zones	Not required	Restorative margin <3 mm apical to mucosal crest	Restorative margin >3 mm apical to mucosal crest
Loading Protocol	To date immediate restoration and loading procedures are lacking scientific documentation	Conventional or early loading		Immediate loading
Materials/Manufacture	Materials and techniques used in the manufacture of definitive prostheses	Resin-based materials ± metal reinforcement	Porcelain fused to metal	
Maintenance Needs	Anticipated maintenance needs based on patient presentation and the planned prosthesis	Low	Moderate	High

3.4.1   General Dental Health

The health status of the oral cavity will have an impact on the degree of difficulty of the implant restorative treatment. The presence of active dental disease has the potential to complicate treatment, and as a general rule, such conditions should be addressed prior to implant therapy.

Occasionally, it is an advantage to be able to modify the shape or appearance of a tooth adjacent to an implant restoration. If such teeth are unrestored and healthy, such treatments are undesirable, and consequently complicate the treatment. If they are restored, modifications are much more readily undertaken.

Implants replacing teeth that have been lost as a consequence of periodontal disease (Baelum and Ellegaard 2004, Karoussis et al. 2003) or occlusal parafunction (Brägger et al. 2001) have greater potential for complications and failure. A history of these issues should alert treating dentists to these risks.

3.4.2   Restorative Volume

The space available for implant restorations will have an impact on the type of restorations that are planned. Generally, whether there is sufficient vertical space for abutments, attachments, and restorative materials will have the most impact on planning, followed by the mesio-distal space available for tooth placement (Martin et al. 2007). If either of these dimensions is restricted to such a degree that implant treatment cannot achieve a functional and/or esthetically acceptable restoration, adjunctive treatments will be necessary. Alternatively, other prosthetic options will need to be employed. Only rarely will restrictions in the oro-facial dimension become apparent, usually in cases where phonetics is compromised by restoration bulk in this dimension.

3.4.3 Volume of the Edentulous Saddle

The dimensions of the edentulous ridge will normally influence the surgical phase of treatment more than the restorative phase. However, where prosthetic replacement of hard and soft tissues is necessary for esthetic or phonetic reasons, this may add an increased level of difficulty to implant treatments.

3.4.4 Occlusion

The patient's occlusal scheme, and the extent to which the implant restoration will be involved in this scheme, will affect the degree of difficulty of implant restoration. This may, in turn, influence the likelihood of complications to the final restoration. Implant restorations that are protected by anterior guidance, but not involved in developing that guidance, will likely have fewer complications from an occlusal point of view than those in group-function situations. Additionally, the presence of an occlusal parafunctional habit in a patient is likely to result in more complications for an implant restoration in terms of screw loosening, abutment or screw fracture, and fracture of the veneering material (Brägger et al. 2001).

3.4.5 Provisional Restorations

Where necessary during the healing phase of implant therapy, interim tooth replacements can add to the difficulty of treatment. This is often most problematic in the fully edentulous case, where interim dentures can place uncontrolled loads on healing implants, increasing the risk of early failure. Care must be taken to ensure that interim tooth replacements do not impinge on healing implants during the critical early healing phase.

Implant-borne provisional restorations are often indicated as a means of developing the esthetic "transition zone"; that is, the development of a restoration emergence profile that mimics that of a natural tooth (Figures 1 to 3). Where these restorations are needed, the depth of placement of the implant shoulder below the mucosal margin will have the most significant effect on the degree of difficulty of the procedure.

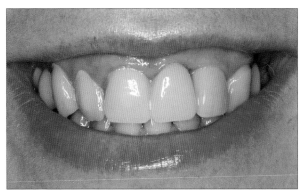

Figure 1.   Facial view of provisional restoration in place.

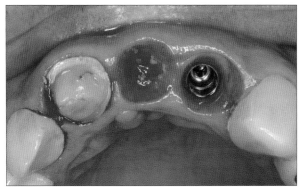

Figure 2.   The provisional bridge has been used to develop the transition zone for the ovate pontic in the 21 site, and the implant crown in the 22 site.

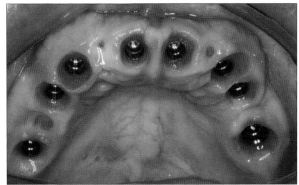

Figure 3.   Provisional bridges have been used to develop the mucosal contours surrounding implant restorations in a full-arch replacement case.

3.4.6   Loading Protocol

When and how implants are loaded by restorations will have an impact on the level of difficulty of the restorative treatment. It should be noted that at present, there is a paucity of evidence to support immediate loading as a routine procedure, except in specific indications in the edentulous mandible (Cochran et al. 2004). Consequently, conventional (healing time of > 3 months) and early (healing time < 3 months but > 2 days) loading will likely be more straightforward than loading in which a provisional or definitive restoration is placed within 48 hours of implant placement – so-called *immediate loading*. The immediate loading protocol is a more difficult technical procedure, and requires greater coordination between the surgeon, restorative dentist, and dental laboratory.

3.4.7   Restorative Materials and Manufacturing Technique

The type of restoration planned for a site, and the materials used to manufacture the restoration, will determine the complexity and difficulty of the treatment procedure.

Here, too, the span of the restoration will have an effect. Resin-based restorative materials, placed over simple metal frameworks, can result in restorations that are easier to make and less prone to distortion (Ortorp and Jemt 2006). In contrast, the porcelain fused to metal technique risks distortion during manufacture, especially over long spans (Bridger and Nicholls 1981, Zervas et al. 1999). This, in turn, may introduce stresses in the restoration due to lack of passive fit. Complications may only become apparent some time after the restoration has been placed. At the very least, this can result in delamination of the porcelain veneering material, which can occur some time after restoration placement.

3.4.8   Maintenance Needs

The need for restoration maintenance should be assessed during the planning of an implant treatment. The span length of the planned restoration, the presence of occlusal parafunction, the restorative technique that is planned, and the dentist's preferences will all impact on this assessment. Generally, more complex restorations will be associated with higher maintenance needs.

3.5 Application

A. Dawson, S. Chen

All of the modifiers discussed above have the potential to be actively considered in an individual implant treatment case. They should be considered in the assessment and planning phases of treatment, and contingency plans should be developed to manage these issues where they have an effect on treatment.

In the following chapters, surgical and restorative issues related to determining normative and specific classifications will be discussed, and modifying factors for various case types will be tabulated. Readers wishing to determine a classification of *Straightforward*, *Advanced* or *Complex* for a specific case can match the specific features of their case with the descriptors outlined in these tables. The SAC Classification for their case will be the level that best matches the factors related to that case.

4 <u>Classification of Surgical Cases</u>

4.1   Principles of Surgical Classification

S. Chen, D. Buser, L. Cordaro

The application of the SAC Classification to surgical cases will follow the general guidelines outlined below. These guidelines will assist in generating the normative classification of a surgical case type. The influence of modifying factors on these case types will be discussed within this chapter.

The case types have been categorized into three groups. The first two groups are distinguished by whether the cases occur in sites of high or low esthetic risk. Within the two groups, cases are sub-categorized into single tooth replacements, short edentulous spaces of up to three teeth using two implants, extended edentulous spaces of more than three teeth in which three or more implants are to be used, and fully edentulous arches. The third group represents implants placed into sockets at the time of tooth extraction, also referred to as immediate implants, or Type 1 placement (Hämmerle et al. 2004). Implants placed in-

to extraction sockets are characterized by specific hard and soft tissue factors, and have therefore been grouped separately.

4.1.1   General Criteria

Surgical cases may be classified as *Straightforward, Advanced* or *Complex* according to the following general criteria:

Straightforward

- The surgical process is anticipated to be uncomplicated, with minimal surgical risk.
- The anatomical risks are minimal.
- Minimal post-operative complications are anticipated.
- There is minimal esthetic risk.

Advanced

- The surgical process is anticipated to be more demanding.
- Proximity to important anatomical structures is likely to increase the difficulty of implant placement.
- There is an increased risk of postoperative complications.
- There is a moderate to high esthetic risk.

Complex

- The surgical process is anticipated to be complicated.
- Proximity to important anatomical structures heightens the difficulty and risk of implant placement.
- Surgical demands on the clinician and ancillary staff are high.
- There is a high risk of surgical complications.
- There is a high esthetic risk.

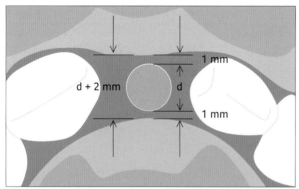

Figure 1.   Schematic representation of the minimum oro-facial width of the bone required to place an implant. The oro-facial width of the bone should be at least 2 mm more than the core diameter of the implant (d + 2 mm, where d = diameter of implant). Provided that the implant is placed in the center of the ridge, this will provide at least 1 mm thickness of bone on the oral and facial aspects of the implant.

4.1.2   Site-Specific Criteria

In addition to the general criteria above, the following site-specific factors were considered for each case type:

Bone volume. This relates to whether there is sufficient bone volume to place an implant or implants in the correct restoratively determined position, without the need for adjunctive augmentation procedures.

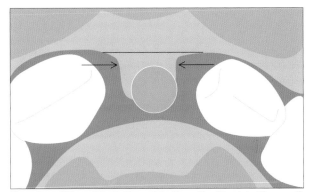

Figure 2a. If the anticipated bone defect has at least two intact bone walls (arrows) and the implant is placed within the confines of the ridge (outer limit of the ridge on the facial aspect is denoted by the line), then the defect is amenable to a bone augmentation procedure simultaneous with implant placement.

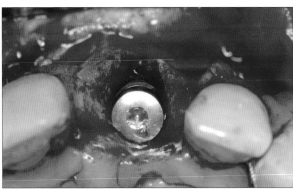

Figure 2b. Occlusal view of an implant in an extraction socket that has lost the facial bone wall. The residual defect has two bone walls remaining on the mesial and distal aspects. The implant is positioned well within the contour of the ridge. A simultaneous bone augmentation procedure may be carried out under these clinical conditions.

- As a general principle, there should be a minimum oro-facial or horizontal bone dimension to maintain at least 1 mm of bone thickness on the facial and oral aspects (Buser et al. 2000). This minimum requirement is depicted in Figure 1.

Core diameter of the implant + 2 mm (to provide 1 mm thickness of facial and oral bone)

Taking into consideration the dimensional differences between commercially available implant systems, the following minimum horizontal bone dimensions are recommended (Table 1):

Narrow diameter implants (diameter range 3.0 to 3.5 mm) – Horizontal bone dimension 5.0 to 5.5 mm

Standard diameter implants (diameter range 3.5 to 4.5 mm) – Horizontal bone dimension 5.5 to 6.5 mm

Wide diameter implants (diameter range 4.5 to 6.0 mm) – Horizontal bone dimension 6.5 to 8.0 mm

- If the preoperative examination determines that the anticipated peri-implant defect will present with at least two bone walls, a simultaneous bone augmentation procedure may be carried out (Figures 2a and 2b). Care should be taken to ensure that the facial surface of the implant does not extend beyond the facial contour of the ridge (Figure 3). If this occurs, the demands on the surgeon to maintain space and to stabilize bone grafts and/or substitutes and barrier membranes increases.

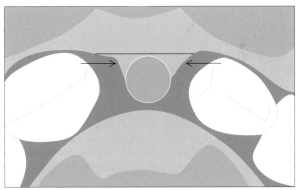

Figure 3. In this example, the bone defect presents with two intact bone walls (arrows). However, the implant is close to the facial limit of the alveolar ridge (line), as determined by the position of the intact bone on adjacent teeth. A simultaneous bone augmentation procedure may be considered; however, there will be greater demands on the surgeon to maintain space and to stabilize grafting materials and barrier membranes, and there is a risk of a less favorable regenerative outcome.

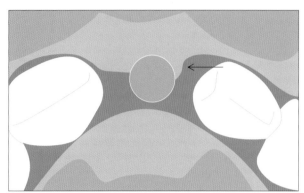

Figure 4.   If the anticipated bone defect has only one wall (arrow), then bone augmentation procedures simultaneous with implant placement are not predictable. In these situations, a staged approach is recommended, i.e., the ridge should be augmented as a first step and the implant placed some time later as a second procedure.

- If the anticipated defect presents as a one-wall defect (Figure 4), a staged bone augmentation approach is recommended. Simultaneous grafting or ridge expansion techniques used for one-wall or no-wall defects should be regarded as *Complex* procedures.

Table 1. Recommended Minimum Oro-facial or Horizontal Bone Width for Implants of Different Dimensions.

Implant Size	Core Diameter* Range (mm)	Minimum Horizontal Bone Dimension (mm)
Narrow diameter implants	3.0 to 3.5	5.0 to 5.5
Standard diameter implants	3.5 to 4.5	5.5 to 6.5
Wide diameter implants	4.5 to 6.0	6.5 to 8.0

* The table refers to the dimensions of the endosseous part of the implant and not the dimensions of the implant shoulder or restorative platform (which may vary depending upon the system and design of the implant).

The core diameter of the implant refers to the diameter of the body of the endosseous part of the implant, and excludes the outer dimensions of the implant threads (if present)

Anatomic risk. This relates to the likely involvement of adjacent roots, neurovascular structures, and the maxillary sinus or nasal cavity, and to perforation of the cortical bone. The anatomic risk at a donor site should also be considered.

Esthetic risk. This relates to the likelihood of pre-existing conditions or hard and soft tissue complications causing adverse esthetic outcomes. In sites of esthetic importance, there is an increased demand for adjunctive hard and soft tissue augmentation procedures and a high level of surgical skill to achieve predictable esthetic outcomes. Modifying factors for the esthetic risk include tissue biotype, lip line at smile, existing bone defects, and patient expectations. For the purpose of the classification, the regions of esthetic priority have been limited to maxillary anterior and premolars sites. It should be recognized that other sites may have esthetic importance depending upon the clinical case.

Complexity. This relates to the perceived difficulty of the planned surgical procedure. The difficulty of a surgical procedure is increased by:

- Management of sites with minimal keratinized mucosa and vestibular depth.
- Immediate placements or ridge preservation procedures.

- Other interventions, including orthodontic tooth movement for site preparation, distraction osteogenesis, ridge splitting or expansion techniques, flapless procedures, and navigational surgery.
- Adjunctive hard and soft tissue grafting procedures performed prior to or at the time of implant placement or as additional procedures after implants have been placed.
- Extra-oral bone harvesting procedures which are considered *Complex* due to high surgical demands on the clinician and ancillary staff.

Complications. All surgical procedures carry a risk of complications with short- and long-term consequences.

Risk of complications: This refers to the likely risk of a complication as a result of the surgical procedure, including donor site morbidity. This also refers to the likely risk of the implant being incorrectly positioned due to pre-existing conditions, or hard and soft tissue complications.

Consequences of complications: The complication may have the following consequences:

- The complication makes the surgical and subsequent restorative process more difficult, but does not have any effect on the outcome.
- The complication results in a sub-optimal outcome which does not reduce the survival of the resulting restoration, but the result falls short of accepted ideals in one or more areas.
- The complication compromises the outcome to a level where long-term success or stability of the implant and final restoration are diminished.
- The complication jeopardizes the success of the whole procedure.

Implants in extraction sockets. Implants may be placed into extraction sockets at the time of tooth extraction (Type 1, or immediate placement) or following soft tissue healing (Type 2, or early placement).

Peri-implant defects with a horizontal component may be augmented as a simultaneous procedure if socket walls are intact or if only the facial wall has been damaged or lost. When two or more walls are missing or a vertical deficiency exists, a staged approach should be considered.

4.1.3   Classification Tables

The classification of surgical case types is presented in the following sections.

The normative classifications assigned refer only to standard presentations of the case type. As previously discussed, modifying factors may alter the normative classification and must be considered when making a final determination of the level of difficulty for the individual case. For the purpose of the classification and for simplification of the tables, esthetic sites are regarded as those in the anterior maxilla. Although upper posterior and all lower sites have been classified in the tables as non-esthetic regions, each case must be determined on its own merits depending upon the presentation of the case and the patient's dental display during normal function and smiling.

It is not the purpose of this classification to list all the possible combinations of surgical procedures that may be required for a particular treatment. However, an indication is given of the types of adjunctive procedures that may be required.

4.2 Implants for Restoration of Single Tooth Spaces in Areas of Low Esthetic Risk

S. Chen

Table 1 represents the classification for implants in single tooth spaces in regions of low esthetic risk. In situations in which the anatomic risk is low and bone volume is sufficient to allow an implant to be placed in the correct restorative position, the level of difficulty and risk of complications is determined to be low. The normative classification is *Straightforward*.

When the bone is deficient horizontally but the site is amenable to an augmentation procedure at the time of implant placement, treatment will likely involve the need for bone grafts or substitutes and/or barrier membranes. These adjunctive techniques increase the degree of difficulty of the treatment, resulting in a normative classification of *Advanced*. It should be noted that the risk of complications may be low for small peri-implant defects, but increases with the size of the defect. If autogenous bone is harvested from a secondary site, donor site morbidity may be an additional complication.

If the site is deficient horizontally to a degree that bone augmentation is required prior to implant placement, the need for horizontal bone augmentation at sites with a lack of supporting bone walls significantly increases the level of difficulty of the treatment. Techniques for lateral bone augmentation may require combinations of autogenous bone grafts (block and/or particulate) or bone substitutes, tenting mechanisms for space maintenance, or barrier membranes (resorbable, non-resorbable and/or reinforced), depending upon operator preference. The level of difficulty is high, with a moderate risk of complications. The normative classification is *Complex* for this case type.

In situations in which there is a lack of sufficient bone height, either due to bone resorption or proximity to important anatomical structures, procedures for increasing the height of bone need to be undertaken. These procedures include onlay bone grafts, vertical guided bone regeneration (GBR), sinus floor augmentation, distraction osteogenesis, and nerve lateralization. In most cases, horizontal augmentation of the deficient site is needed. These procedures have a high level of difficulty and should only be performed by experienced surgeons. There is an elevated risk of involvement of important anatomical structures and of postoperative complications. For these reasons, the normative classification for this case type is *Complex*.

Table 1. Surgical Classification of Cases in Single-Tooth Spaces in Areas of Low Esthetic Risk.

Areas of Low Esthetic Risk	Case Type: Single Tooth Space					
Risk Assessment					**Normative Classification**	**Notes/Adjunctive Procedures that may be required**
Bone Volume	**Anatomic Risk**	**Esthetic Risk**	**Complexity**	**Risk of Complications**		
Defining Characteristics: One implant						
Sufficient	Low	Low	Low	Low	Straight-forward	
Deficient horizontally, allowing simultaneous augmentation	Low	Low	Moderate	Low	Advanced	Procedures for simultaneous horizontal bone augmentation Low risk of complications for small defects, but risk may increase for larger defects Donor site morbidity
Deficient horizontally, requiring prior grafting	Low	Low	High	Moderate	Complex	Procedures for horizontal bone augmentation Involvement of the mental foramina in the mandible Donor site morbidity
Deficient vertically	High	Low	High	High	Complex	Procedures for vertical and/or horizontal bone augmentation Involvement of the mental foramina in the mandible Procedures for sinus floor grafting Risk to adjacent teeth with some vertical augmentation procedures Donor site morbidity

4.2.1 Clinical Case – Missing Lower Left Premolar and Molar

This is a case of a missing lower left second premolar (35) and first molar (36) in a healthy 28-year-old male patient (Figure 1). Although two teeth were missing, clinical examination showed 11 mm of mesio-distal space and 6 mm of vertical space from the mucosa to the opposing dentition. Slight supra-eruption of the upper left second premolar (25) was evident. The patient presented with good oral hygiene, and was dentally and periodontally healthy. A panoramic radiograph showed the presence of the mental foramen 12 to 14 mm from the crest of the ridge

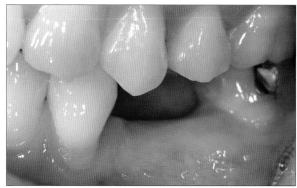

Figure 1. Facial view of missing lower left first molar (tooth 36) showing sufficient mesio-distal space and adequate vertical clearance for implant therapy.

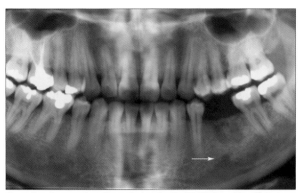

Figure 2.   Panoramic radiograph showing the 35, 36 site, with sufficient vertical bone height superior to the mandibular canal. Note the location of the mental foramen (arrow).

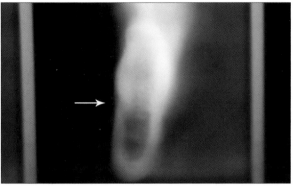

Figure 3.   Plain-film tomogram of the 35, 36 site showing sufficient horizontal bone width and a minimal lingual concavity of the ridge. Note the position of the mental foramen (arrow).

(Figure 2). A plain film tomographic view showed a ridge of 7 to 8 mm in horizontal dimension, and the presence of a minimal lingual concavity in the mandible (Figure 3). The treatment plan was to place a single wide-diameter implant to support a single crown.

The bone volume was sufficient to place an implant with minimal anatomic risk. The procedure was determined to have a relatively low level of difficulty, with a low risk of operative and postoperative complications. The surgical SAC Classification was therefore determined to be *Straightforward* (Table 2).

Table 2. Surgical SAC Classification for the Case of a Missing Lower Left Premolar and Molar to be Restored with a Single Implant-Supported Restoration.

General Factors	Assessment	Notes
Medical contraindications	None	
Smoking habit	None	
Growth considerations	None	
Site Factors	**Assessment**	**Notes**
Bone volume	Sufficient	
Anatomic risk	Low	Mental foramen 12 to 14 mm from ridge crest Minimal risk of perforating the lingual cortex
Esthetic risk	Low	
Complexity	Low	Sufficient mouth-opening to provide adequate surgical access Sufficient bone volume to allow implant placement without the need for adjunctive bone augmentation procedures.
Risk of complications	Low	Risk of complications will be low with insertion of an implant 10 mm in length
Loading protocol	Early	The plan was to restore the implant 6 to 8 weeks after placement
SAC Classification	Straightforward	

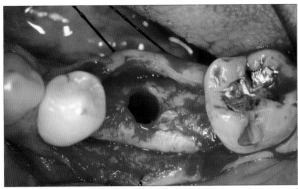

Figure 4. Intra-operative view of the osteotomy, showing maintenance of sufficient thickness of the facial and oral bone walls.

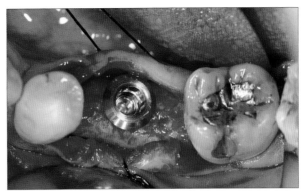

Figure 5. Intra-operative view of the implant in place.

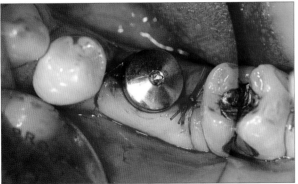

Figure 6. A healing cap was attached to the implant and the flaps were closed with interrupted sutures.

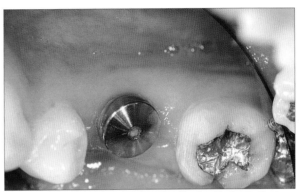

Figure 7. Clinical situation after six weeks of healing. The implant had successfully integrated.

Following reflection of full-thickness facial and oral flaps, the ridge was exposed and the horizontal width of bone was confirmed (Figure 4). The facial and oral surfaces of the ridge were explored to confirm that there were no defects or concavities. A 10 mm Straumann SLA implant (Straumann Implant System, Straumann AG, Basel, Switzerland) with a wide neck (6.5 mm) and 4.8 mm body was placed (Figure 5). A bone wall thickness of 1 mm was maintained on both the facial and oral surfaces of the implant. A healing cap was then attached to the implant and the flaps were closed with interrupted sutures (Figure 6). Six weeks later, the implant had successfully integrated (Figures 7 and 8) and was subsequently restored with a cement-retained PFM crown.

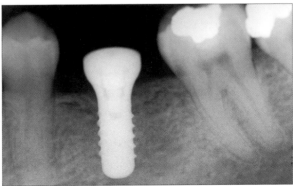

Figure 8. Periapical radiograph of the implant six weeks after placement.

4.3 Implants for Restoration of Short Edentulous Spaces in Areas of Low Esthetic Risk

D. Buser

Table 1 summarizes the classification for the surgical placement of implants in short edentulous spaces in areas of low esthetic risk. These cases will be limited to the replacement of up to three teeth supported by one or two implants. When the anatomic risk is low and bone volume is sufficient to allow implants to be placed in the correct restorative position, the level of difficulty and risk of complications is low. The normative classification is *Straightforward*.

When the bone is deficient horizontally but the defect allows implant placement with a simultaneous bone augmentation procedure, treatment will usually involve the need for bone grafts or substitutes and/or barrier membranes. These additional procedures increase the degree of difficulty of the treatment, and are assigned a normative classification of *Advanced*. Although the risk of complications may be low for small peri-implant defects, the risk increases correspondingly with an increase in the size of the defect. If autogenous bone is harvested from a secondary site, donor site morbidity may be an additional complication.

If the site is deficient horizontally and the peri-implant defect is expected to have fewer than two intact bone walls, a staged approach is strongly recommended. The need for horizontal bone augmentation at sites with a lack of supporting bone walls significantly increases the level of difficulty for the surgeon. Techniques for horizontal bone augmentation may require various combinations of autogenous bone grafts or bone substitutes, tenting mechanisms for space maintenance, and barrier membranes, depending upon the clinical indication and the surgeon's preference. These procedures require the surgeon to be well-trained and experienced. Implants can only be placed following a successful outcome with the initial augmentation procedure. The level of difficulty is therefore regarded as high, with a moderate risk of complications. The normative classification is *Complex* for this case type.

At sites that lack sufficient bone height either due to resorptive processes or due to proximity to important anatomical structures, procedures for increasing the height of bone need to be undertaken. These procedures include onlay bone grafts and vertical guided bone regeneration. In most cases, there is a concomitant need for horizontal augmentation of the deficient site. These procedures have a high level of difficulty and carry a high risk of involvement of important anatomical structures and of postoperative complications. The normative classification is *Complex*.

Table 1. Surgical Classification of Cases in Short Edentulous Spaces in Areas Low Esthetic Risk.

Areas of Low Esthetic Risk	Case Type: Short Edentulous Space						
Risk Assessment						Normative Classification	Notes/Adjunctive Procedures that may be required
Bone Volume	Anatomic Risk	Esthetic Risk	Complexity	Risk of Complications			
Defining Characteristics: Two implants and up to 3 teeth replaced							
Sufficient	Low	Low	Low	Low		Straight-forward	
Deficient horizontally, allowing simultaneous grafting	Low	Low	Moderate	Moderate		Advanced	Procedures for simultaneous horizontal bone augmentation Low risk of complications for small defects, but risk may increase for larger defects Donor site morbidity
Deficient horizontally, requiring prior grafting	Low	Low	High	Moderate		Complex	Procedures for horizontal bone augmentation Involvement of the mental foramina in the mandible Donor site morbidity
Deficient vertically and/or horizontally	High	Low	High	High		Complex	Procedures for vertical and/or horizontal bone augmentation Involvement of the mental foramina in the mandible Procedures for sinus floor grafting Risk to adjacent teeth with some vertical augmentation procedures Donor site morbidity

4.3.1 Clinical Case – Missing Lower Left Premolar and Molar

A female patient presented with a loss of retention of a short-span, three-unit fixed dental prosthesis (FDP) in the left mandible due to caries that had undermined the retainer attached to the second premolar. The clinical examination revealed that the root of tooth 35 could not be maintained and had to be removed (Figure 1). In the first molar site, the bone crest was clearly reduced in horizontal width due to non-functional atrophy. The panoramic radiograph showed sufficient bone height in general in

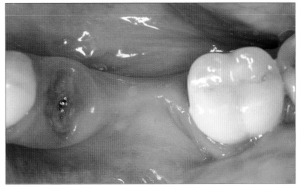

Figure 1.   Occlusal view of the case showing the root of tooth 35.

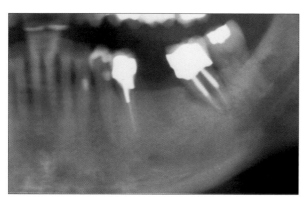

Figure 2.   Panoramic radiograph of the lower left quadrant.

the left mandible (Figure 2). The mental foramen was located slightly distal to the apex of tooth 35. Tooth 37 was clearly tilted mesially and exhibited radiolucency on the mesial aspect. The patient expressed a desire to restore the occlusion in the left mandible with a fixed restoration, if possible without a staged approach. The treatment plan was to extract the roots of tooth 35 and tooth 37, and to use the concept of early implant placement to keep the risk of complications low. Implants would be placed in the 35 and 37 sites with simultaneous GBR. The implants would support a three-unit FDP.

The preoperative assessment indicated that there was sufficient bone width and height in both the proposed implant sites (35 and 37). However, an extraction socket defect was anticipated in the 35 site, with possible damage to the facial bone wall. The anatomic risk was low, but care would need to be taken at the time of surgery to avoid injury to the mental nerve. The level of difficulty was determined to be high due to the need for a simultaneous GBR procedure with primary wound closure. The risk of complications with the GBR procedure was regarded as low. The risk of damage to the mental nerve was also judged to be low with careful flap elevation and protection of the mental nerve throughout the procedure. The surgical SAC Classification was determined to be *Advanced* (Table 2).

Table 2. Surgical SAC Classification for the Case with a Missing Lower Left Premolar and Molar.

General Factors	Assessment	Notes
Medical contraindications	None	
Smoking habit	None	
Growth considerations	None	
Site Factors	**Assessment**	**Notes**
Bone volume in sites 35 and 37	Sufficient in width, but extraction socket defect in area 35	Two-wall defect in area 35 Standard placement in area 37
Anatomic risk	Low	Mental foramen is located in between the two future implant positions
Esthetic risk	Low	
Complexity	Moderate	Simultaneous GBR procedure for implant 35
Risk of complications	Low	Risk of complications will be low with simultaneous GBR procedure Mental nerve may be involved with flap reflection and needs to be protected throughout the procedure
Loading protocol	Early	
SAC Classification	Advanced	

The roots of teeth 35 and 37 were then extracted (Figure 3). Following a soft tissue healing period of 6 weeks (Figure 4), implant placement was planned for the extraction socket defect in area 35 and slightly mesial to the extraction socket defect in area 37 (Figure 5). It was anticipated that the 35 site would have a defect on the facial aspect, with two intact bone walls. Thus implant placement with a simultaneous GBR procedure was possible in this site, which was given a normative classification of Advanced. In area 37, standard implant placement was possible with non-submerged healing (Figure 6). Following an uneventful healing period of 8 weeks, the 35 implant was exposed with a punch technique and a healing cap was attached. Restorative procedures commenced soon after this, and two weeks later an implant-borne three-unit FDP was inserted (Figure 7 and 8).

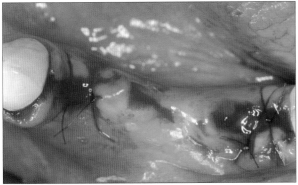

Figure 3.   Occlusal view of the surgical sites immediately following extraction of the roots of tooth 35 and tooth 37.

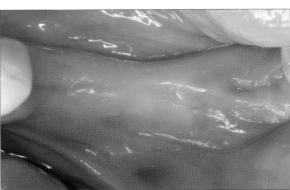

Figure 4.   Occlusal view of the ridge six weeks following extraction of the teeth.

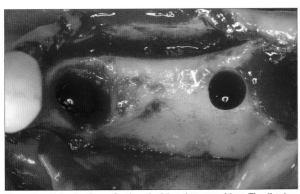

Figure 5.   Following flap reflection, the 35 socket was evident. The distal osteotomy was prepared slightly mesial to the 37 socket.

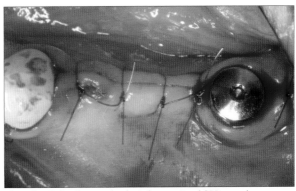

Figure 6.   A simultaneous implant placement and GBR procedure was performed in the 35 site, with primary closure of the flap. In the 37 site, standard placement was performed using a non-submerged healing protocol.

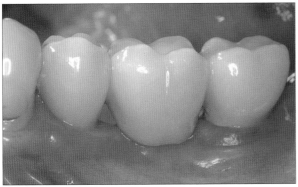

Figure 7.   Facial view of the implant-borne three-unit FDP.

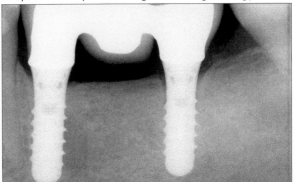

Figure 8.   Radiographic view of the implants and completed FDP.

4.4 Implants for Restoration of Extended Edentulous Spaces in Areas of Low Esthetic Risk

L. Cordaro

Table 1 outlines the classification for implant surgical procedures aimed to restore extended edentulous spaces in regions of low esthetic risk. An extended edentulous space is defined as a site where more than three teeth are missing and more than two implants are needed to support a FDP. In situations in which the anatomic and esthetic risks are low and bone volume is sufficient to allow implants of appropriate dimensions to be placed in the correct restorative position, the procedure is considered to be *Straightforward*. The level of complexity is deemed to be moderate due to the increased number of implants placed and demands on the surgeon to maintain a proper relative alignment and position of the implants. The risk of complications is regarded as low.

When a similar situation involves an alveolar segment with reduced bone width that can be augmented at the time of implant placement, the normative classification is *Advanced*. Both the anatomical and surgical risks are moderate due to the bone augmentation procedures needed at the time of implant placement. These procedures usually involve the use of grafts with autogenous bone or bone substitutes that may require protection during healing with either resorbable or non-resorbable membranes. The esthetic risk is low and the complexity is moderate.

A different normative classification is assigned to extended edentulous spans in non-esthetic sites when the horizontal bone deficiency needs to be corrected before implant placement in a separate surgical procedure. Reconstructive procedures include block bone grafts or guided bone regeneration with combinations of autogenous bone or bone substitutes and resorbable, non-resorbable, or reinforced barrier membranes. The complexity of the procedure is high due to the increased demands on the surgeon and the need for multiple surgical procedures. It should be noted that the possibility of placing implants in a second procedure is contingent upon successful horizontal augmentation of the ridge in the first instance. If the outcome of bone augmentation is sub-optimal, the subsequent implant placements may be compromised. The esthetic risk is low but the anatomical risk and the risk of complications are moderate. This case type has a normative classification of *Complex*.

In cases that show a vertical alveolar deficiency with or without an associated horizontal defect, the surgical procedure should be considered *Complex*. In these cases, the need for very demanding reconstructive procedures prior to or at the time of implant placement is usually associated with a high anatomical risk and a high risk of complications and failures. These factors increase the complexity of the procedure to a high level. When a vertical augmentation is needed in mandibular posterior sites, the procedure must be considered very challenging, even for the very experienced surgeon.

Table 1. Surgical Classification of Cases in Extended Edentulous Spaces in Areas of Low Esthetic Risk.

Areas of Low Esthetic Risk	Case Type: Extended Edentulous Space					
Risk Assessment					Normative Classification	Notes/Adjunctive Procedures that may be required
Bone Volume	Anatomic Risk	Esthetic Risk	Complexity	Risk of Complications	Normative Classification	Notes/Adjunctive Procedures that may be required
Defining Characteristics: More than 2 implants, span of more than 3 teeth						
Sufficient	Low	Low	Moderate	Low	Straight-forward	None
Deficient horizontally, allowing simultaneous grafting	Moderate	Low	Moderate	Moderate	Advanced	Procedures for simultaneous horizontal bone augmentation Low risk of complications for small defects, but risk may increase for larger defects Involvement of the mental foramina in the mandible Donor site morbidity
Deficient horizontally, requiring prior grafting	Moderate	Low	High	Moderate	Complex	Procedures for horizontal bone augmentation Involvement of the mental foramina in the mandible Donor site morbidity
Deficient vertically, with or without a horizontal defect	High	Low	High	High	Complex	Risk to adjacent teeth Procedures for vertical and/or horizontal bone augmentation Involvement of the mental foramen and inferior alveolar nerve in the mandible Procedures for sinus floor grafting Donor site morbidity

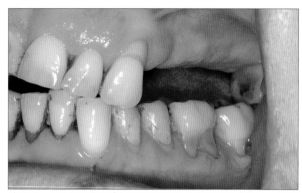

Figure 1.   Intraoral view of the extended edentulous space in the upper left posterior sextant. Teeth 24, 25, 26 and 27 were missing.

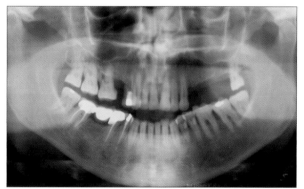

Figure 2.   Panoramic radiograph of the case, showing missing teeth in the upper left posterior sextant.

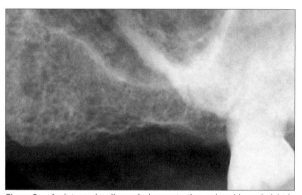

Figure 3.   An intraoral radiograph demonstrating reduced bone height in the first and second molar sites.

4.4.1   Clinical Case – Four Missing Posterior Teeth in the Upper Left Quadrant

A 58-year-old woman with an extended edentulous space in the upper left quadrant requested a fixed rehabilitation (Figure 1). No general health problems were present, and acceptable oral hygiene was maintained. An anterior open bite was evident and a noticeable functional impairment was present. Panoramic and intra-oral radiographs demonstrated reduced bone height in the region of the first and second molars (Figures 2 and 3). The treatment plan was to augment the height of bone in the posterior maxilla by elevating the floor of the maxillary sinus and placing a synthetic bone graft. Following maturation of the graft, it was planned to insert three implants to support a four-unit FDP. Implants were planned to be placed in the first premolar and first and second molar sites. In this way, no cantilever units would be included in the prosthesis, and a better esthetic result was anticipated at the premolar sites by avoiding adjacent implants.

The pre-operative assessment confirmed sufficient horizontal bone dimension but reduced vertical bone dimension in the molar region. Due to involvement of the maxillary sinus, the anatomic risk was high. The esthetic risk was assessed to be moderate, as the upper premolar teeth were visible in the patient's smile. As multiple procedures were planned and surgical technical demands associated with the augmentation of the sinus floor were significant, the level of complexity was regarded as high. However, through staging of the treatment, any complications associated with the sinus floor augmentation procedure would be independent of the implants subsequently placed. Thus, the risk of complications and the sequelae of any complications were regarded as only moderate. The surgical SAC Classification was assessed as *Complex* (Table 2).

Table 2. Surgical SAC Classification for the Case of Four Missing Posterior Teeth in the Upper Left Quadrant.

General Factors	Assessment	Notes
Medical contraindications	None	
Smoking habit	None	
Growth considerations	None	
Site Factors	**Assessment**	**Notes**
Bone volume	Adequate in width	Vertical deficiency in the first and second molar sites Sinus floor augmentation required
Anatomic risk	High	Involvement of the maxillary sinus
Esthetic risk	Moderate	Posterior edentulous space Upper premolar teeth visible in the patient's smile.
Complexity	High	A staged approach is required. Technical demands associated with the sinus augmentation procedure Implants may only be placed in the molar sites following a successful outcome of the initial sinus augmentation procedure.
Risk of complications	Moderate	Risk of perioperative and postoperative complications associated with the sinus floor augmentation procedure
Loading protocol	Early	
SAC Classification	Complex	

Augmentation of the floor of the sinus was planned with a synthetic bone substitute to avoid the need for harvesting autogenous bone. Since only the reconstructive phase was planned during the first surgical step, access to the lateral sinus wall was obtained following elevation of a mucoperiosteal flap with vertical releasing incisions that did not involve the marginal tissues of the canine. Once the elevation of the sinus mucosa was performed, a biphasic calcium phosphate material (Straumann Bone Ceramic, Straumann AG, Basel, Switzerland) was applied in the defect as an inlay graft (Figures 4 to 6). Four months lat-

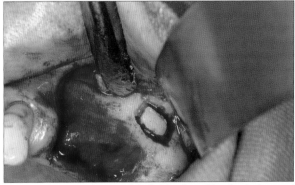

Figure 4. Intraoperative view of the facial surface of the alveolar bone and the outline of the window into the maxillary sinus.

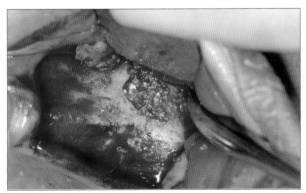

Figure 5. Intraoperative view of the lateral window following placement of the graft.

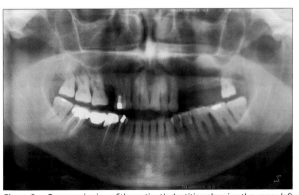

Figure 6. Panoramic view of the patient's dentition showing the upper left posterior sextant after sinus floor elevation.

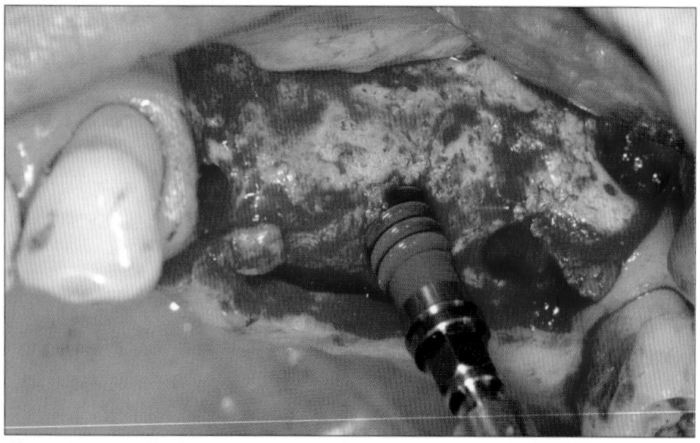

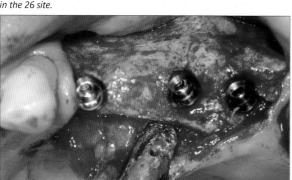

Figure 7.   Surgical re-entry was performed four months later. The intraoperative view shows the three osteotomy sites and an implant being inserted in the 26 site.

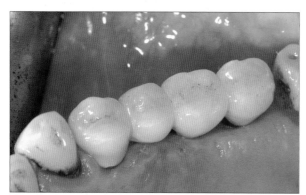

Figure 8.   The intraoperative occlusal view shows adequate bone width. The three implants were installed in the planned locations.

er, two wide-body SLActive implants (Straumann Implant System, Straumann AG, Basel, Switzerland) with a 4.8 mm diameter of the neck and of the implant body were inserted in the molar sites. One standard SLActive implant was inserted in the region of the first premolar (Figures 7 and 8). All implants were 10 mm in length. Implant location and axial orientation were verified with a surgical stent. After four months the implants were restored with a four-unit porcelain-fused-to-metal FDP. The occlusal view shows the reduced oro-facial dimensions of the prosthesis (Figures 9 and 10). The final radiographs demonstrate the effective reconstruction of the deficient ridge and stable marginal bone levels (Figures 11 and 12).

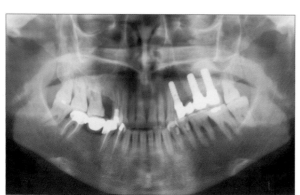

Figure 9.   Intraoral occlusal view of the completed four-unit FDP.

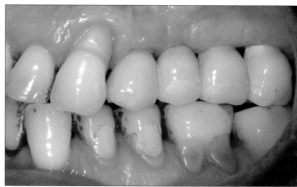

Figure 10.   Intraoral facial view of the completed four-unit FDP.

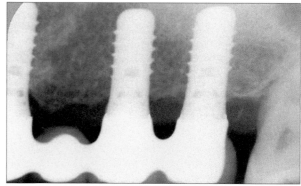

Figure 11.   Panoramic radiograph of the completed case.

Figure 12.   Periapical radiograph of the completed case, showing stable crestal bone.

4.5 Implants for an Implant-supported Denture or a Full-arch Fixed Dental Prosthesis in the Edentulous Mandible

D. Buser

Table 1 represents the classification for implant procedures in the edentulous mandible, which in most cases represents an indication for implant therapy with low esthetic risk.

In general, the treatment options may be differentiated into two groups:

- 2 to 4 implants being placed in the anterior mandible between the mental foramina, or
- 6 to 8 implants being placed in the entire mandible.

In posterior implant sites distal to the mental foramina, bone height is often reduced to the extent that implant placement may be difficult or impossible. Thus, implants placed between the mental foramina are often used to stabilize removable full dentures, and is a procedure that is well documented in the literature (Feine et al. 2002). The placement of two implants in the canine region in patients with sufficient bone volume has a normative classification of *Straightforward*. This situation has a low anatomic risk, since the mental nerves are fairly distant from both implant sites.

The normative classification is revised to *Advanced* if the placement of two implants has to be combined with simultaneous bone augmentation due to localized bone defects. The classification is also regarded as *Advanced* if three to four implants in the inter-foraminal region or more than four implants in total (including implant sites distal to the mental foramina) are planned. This *Advanced* classification is due to the increased risk caused by proximity to the mental nerves, and to the increased numbers of implants placed. The demands on the surgeon to maintain proper relative alignment and position of the implants are high.

The normative classification *Complex* is assigned to clinical situations for which more than two implants are placed in sites with localized bone defects that require bone augmentation procedures (either staged or simultaneous). Additionally, adjustment and stabilization of interim removable full dentures after implant surgery or bone augmentation procedures are significant clinical problems. Great care needs to be taken to ensure that the implants are not loaded prematurely, or that the removable prosthesis does not create areas of pressure over the healing mucosa and underlying grafts. For these reasons, patients are often advised not to wear their interim prosthesis during the initial healing phase, a situation which is not always acceptable to patients. To overcome this, provisional implants may be used to support a fixed interim prosthesis. Alternatively, immediate loading protocols (with either fixed or removable prostheses) may be considered when four or more implants can be placed with good initial stability. Immediate loading protocols (using either provisional or the definitive implants) require close coordination with the restorative dentist and the dental laboratory. Implant placement combined with immediate loading in the edentulous mandible is regarded as a *Complex* procedure.

Table 1. Surgical Classification of Cases for Full Arch Replacements in Areas of Low Esthetic Risk.

Areas of Low Esthetic Risk	Case Type: Full Arch – Mandible					
Risk Assessment					**Normative Classification**	**Notes/Adjunctive Procedures that may be required**
Bone Volume	**Anatomic Risk**	**Esthetic Risk**	**Complexity**	**Risk of Complications**		
Defining Characteristics: 2 implants, interforaminal region						
Sufficient	Low	Low	Low	Low	Straight-forward	None
Deficient, but allowing simultaneous bone augmentation	Moderate	Low	Moderate	Moderate	Advanced	Risk of perforation of lingual cortex Procedures for simultaneous horizontal bone augmentation
Defining Characteristics: 3 or 4 implants, interforaminal region						
Sufficient	Moderate	Low	Moderate	Moderate	Advanced	Involvement of the mental foramina
Deficient, but allowing simultaneous or prior bone augmentation	Moderate	Low	High	High	Complex	Risk of mental nerve involvement Risk of perforation of lingual cortex Procedures for simultaneous or prior horizontal bone augmentation
Defining Characteristics: > 4 implants, extending distal to interforaminal region						
Sufficient both in vertical and horizontal dimensions	Moderate	Low	Moderate	Moderate	Advanced	Involvement of the mental foramina
Deficient, but allowing simultaneous or prior bone augmentation	High	Low	High	High	Complex	Risk of mental nerve involvement Risk of perforation of lingual cortex Risk of inferior alveolar nerve involvement Procedures for simultaneous or prior horizontal bone augmentation
Defining Characteristics: 4 or more implants, immediate loading						
Sufficient	Moderate	Low	High	Moderate	Complex	Coordination with restorative practitioners and laboratory technicians

4.5.1 Clinical Case – Implant Placement in an Edentulous Mandible Following Extraction

A 55-year-old male patient presented with a dentition of five remaining teeth in the mandible (Figure 1). Clinical and radiographic examination showed advanced periodontitis for all teeth remaining in the mandible (Figure 2). Thus, it was decided to extract all teeth and immediately place four implants in the anterior mandible to support a bar-type overdenture.

On assessment of the case, it was noted that bone volume in the inter-foraminal region was sufficient to allow implants to be placed. However, a moderate anatomical risk

was identified due to the proximity of the distal implants to the mental foramina. It was anticipated that any peri-implant bone defects would be relatively small following extraction of the teeth and reduction of the alveolar ridges. Thus the need for simultaneous bone augmentation procedures was reduced. The surgical procedure involving tooth extraction, ridge reduction and placement of four implants with good relative alignment, was assessed as having a moderate degree of complexity. It was planned to fabricate and deliver the retentive bar within a few days of implant placement but to defer loading for several weeks. Coordination with the restorative dentist and laboratory technician would therefore be required. A classification of *Advanced* was assigned to this case (Table 2).

Table 2. Surgical SAC Classification for Implant Placement in the Anterior Mandible with an Immediate Loading Protocol.

General Factors	Assessment	Notes
Medical contraindications	None	
Smoking habit	None	
Growth considerations	None	
Site Factors	**Assessment**	**Notes**
Bone volume	Sufficient	Sufficient vertical and horizontal bone dimension to allow implants of a standard diameter to be placed
Anatomic risk	Moderate	The anterior loop of the mental foramina needs to be respected
Esthetic risk	Low	
Complexity	Moderate	Standard implant placement following the flattening of the crest, grafting of remaining extraction socket Placement of four implants with good relative alignment
Risk of complications	Moderate	Risk of complication will be low with insertion of implants 10 mm in length Risk of involvement of the anterior loop of the mental nerves
Loading protocol	Early	Although the retentive bar would be attached to the implants soon after surgery, loading was to be deferred for several weeks
SAC classification	Advanced	

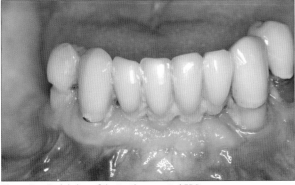

Figure 1.   Facial view of the tooth-supported FDP.

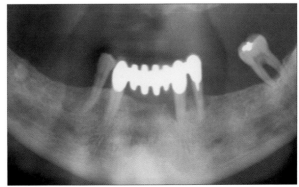

Figure 2.   Panoramic radiograph of the dentition at presentation.

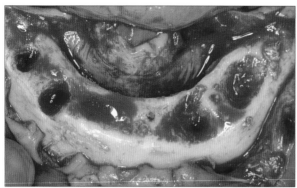

Figure 3. Surgical view of the ridge following extraction of the teeth and flattening of the ridge.

Following extraction of all teeth, the bone crest was flattened by a few millimeters. This reduced the dimensions of the residual root sockets. Four implant sites were selected and the sites prepared (Figure 3). With this approach, all four implant sites did not exhibit peri-implant bone defects, and implants could be placed with a standard placement protocol. The remaining sockets, however, were filled with locally harvested autogenous bone grafts (Figure 4). Following suturing, an impression was taken to fabricate an implant-supported bar (Figure 5). The bar was attached to the implants within 24 hours of surgery, but not loaded (Figure 6). After a healing period

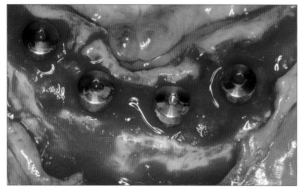

Figure 4. Surgical view of the four implants and grafted extraction sockets.

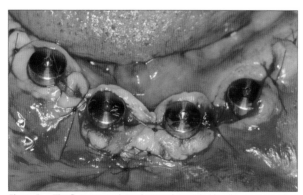

Figure 5. The flaps were adapted around extended healing caps attached to the implants.

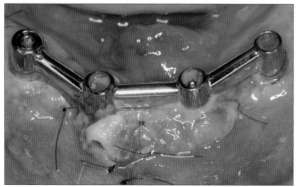

Figure 6. Facial view of the retentive bar attached to the four implants.

of a few weeks, the overdenture was fabricated and issued to the patient. The follow-up at two years demonstrated good peri-implant tissue stability (Figures 7 to 9).

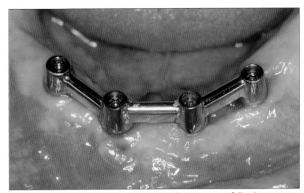

Figure 7.   Facial view of the clinical situation two years following surgery.

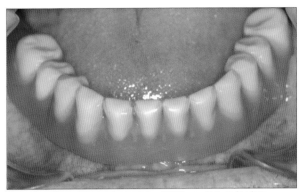

Figure 8.   View of the implant-retained full lower denture in place.

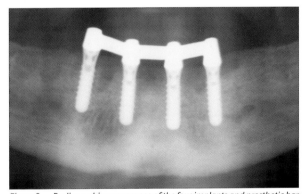

Figure 9.   Radiographic appearance of the four implants and prosthetic bar two years following surgery.

4.6   Implants for Restoration of Single Tooth Spaces in Areas of High Esthetic Risk

L. Cordaro

Table 1 represents the surgical classification for replacement of missing single teeth in regions of high esthetic risk. By definition, any treatment in the esthetic zone involves a risk of esthetic complications. For single tooth replacements, the esthetic outcome depends upon achieving symmetry of tooth form and soft tissue contour with the contralateral natural teeth. In this regard, two factors within the responsibility of the surgeon are critical. First, the implants have to be positioned very precisely from a three-dimensional point of view to allow for an esthetic treatment outcome. To facilitate this, the concept of the *Comfort* and *Danger Zones* was established by the ITI Consensus Conference in 2003 (Buser et al. 2004). Surgical stents are recommended in these situations. Second, management of the hard and soft tissues with appropriate augmentation procedures at the time of surgery is essential. Adjunctive soft tissue grafting procedures may be necessary even in the presence of adequate bone volume.

Table 1. Surgical Classification of Cases for Single-Tooth Spaces in Areas of High Esthetic Risk.

Areas of High Esthetic Risk	Case Type: Single Tooth					
Risk Assessment					**Normative Classification**	**Notes/Adjunctive Procedures that may be required**
Bone Volume	**Anatomic Risk**	**Esthetic Risk**	**Complexity**	**Risk of Complications**		
Defining Characteristics: One implant						
Sufficient	Low	High	Moderate	Moderate	Advanced	Risk of recession at adjacent teeth Adjunctive soft tissue graft
Deficient horizontally, allowing simultaneous grafting	Low	High	Moderate	Moderate	Advanced	Risk of recession at adjacent teeth Adjunctive soft tissue graft Procedures for simultaneous horizontal bone augmentation
Deficient horizontally, requiring prior grafting	Low	High	Moderate	Moderate	Complex	Risk of recession at adjacent teeth Adjunctive soft tissue graft Procedures for horizontal bone augmentation
Deficient vertically and/or horizontally	High	High	High	High	Complex	Risk of recession at adjacent teeth Adjunctive soft tissue graft Procedures for vertical and/or horizontal bone augmentation

Each case must be assessed comprehensively; a systematic approach to esthetic risk assessment is recommended (Martin et al. 2007). Thus, when implants for single tooth replacements are needed in the esthetic zone, the surgical procedure involved must be considered *Advanced* or *Complex*.

If the available volume of bone is sufficient and an implant of adequate dimensions can be inserted in the correct position and angulation, the normative classification is *Advanced*. The anatomical risk may be regarded as low, but the complexity of the procedure and the risk of esthetic complications are moderate due to the requirement for a precise three-dimensional positioning of the implant. This is of paramount importance for the achievement of an esthetically satisfactory final restoration.

For situations in which the available volume is deficient horizontally and conditions allow for bone augmentation at the time of implant placement, the normative classification is still *Advanced*. Usually, simultaneous horizontal augmentation is achieved with guided bone regenerative procedures that involve the use of allogeneic or xenogeneic grafting materials, autogenous bone chips harvested locally, and barrier membranes. Although the anatomical risk is regarded as low, care should be taken to identify possible complications that may arise from proximity to the nasopalatine canal. The complexity and risk of complications are moderate due to the esthetic demands.

When the horizontal bony deficiency must be corrected with a separate surgical procedure in preparation for implant placement, the complexity of the procedure is high, and consequently the entire procedure must be considered *Complex*. A staged approach is recommended in these cases. The augmentation procedures carried out in the first surgical step may involve the use of autologous bone blocks fixed with screws or autogenous bone chips or xenografts in conjunction with either resorbable or non-resorbable barrier membranes. If there is the need for a second surgical site for bone harvesting, the complexity and the risk of complications of the procedure are increased accordingly. In the second surgical step the implant is inserted after removal of barrier membranes or lag screws. In some instances a submerged approach may be used, and a third very simple surgical procedure to uncover the implant shoulder may be necessary.

Vertical bone deficiency in single tooth spaces in the esthetic zone represents one of the most difficult challenges in implant dentistry. A staged approach is used by most surgeons, and involves alveolar reconstruction and implant placement in separate procedures. Vertical reconstruction is usually achieved with GBR or bone grafting procedures, as in treatment for horizontal augmentations.

It should be noted that specific surgical factors may further increase the complexity of the procedure and risk of complications. For example, accurate soft tissue management is necessary to achieve and maintain soft tissue coverage of the reconstructed alveolus during healing. The coronal limits of the bony reconstruction are the interproximal bony peaks of the adjacent teeth, and this must be taken into consideration for a correct treatment plan. For these reasons, cases with vertical deficiency of a single tooth space in the esthetic zone should be considered *Complex*.

4.6.1 Clinical Case – Missing Upper Central Incisor with Horizontal and Vertical Bony Deficiency

This clinical case illustrates the replacement of a failing upper left central incisor (tooth 21) previously treated with endodontic surgery (Figures 1 and 2). The patient was a young female with high esthetic demands who requested replacement with a fixed restoration. She reported recurrent acute infections of the tooth. Her oral hygiene was acceptable.

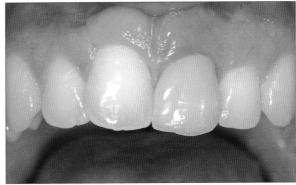

Figure 1.   Facial view of the maxillary anterior teeth. Tooth 21 had a deep pocket on the mid-facial aspect.

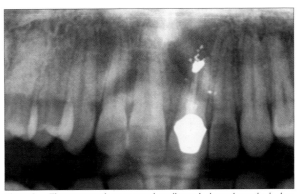

Figure 2.   The preoperative panoramic radiograph showed a periapical radiolucency.

The preoperative analysis revealed a deep pocket on the mid-facial aspect of the tooth, indicating that the facial bone was damaged. A risk assessment determined that the bone volume following tooth extraction was likely to be deficient vertically and horizontally. The anatomic risk was moderate: the thin nature of the soft tissues would require careful surgical management, and there was potential involvement of the nasopalatine canal. The esthetic risk was high due to the location of the site in the esthetic zone, thin tissues that increased the risk of marginal tissue recession, and the patient's high esthetic expectations. This analysis suggested that a staged approach to treatment would be necessary, commencing with tooth extraction, subsequent bone augmentation, and implant placement. Adjunctive soft tissue augmentation was likely to be required. Both the level of complexity and risk of complications were regarded as high. For these reasons, the SAC Classification was *Complex* (Table 2).

Table 2. Surgical SAC Classification for the Case of a Missing Upper Central Incisor with Horizontal and Vertical Bony Deficiency.

General Factors	Assessment	Notes
Medical contraindications	None	
Smoking habit	None	
Growth considerations	None	
Site Factors	**Assessment**	**Notes**
Bone volume	Vertical and horizontal deficiency	Staged approach indicated to optimize the hard and soft tissue outcomes
Anatomic risk	Moderate	Thin tissue biotype requires careful handling at the time of surgery Proximity to the nasopalatine canal may affect ideal three-dimensional position of the implant
Esthetic risk	High	Thin biotype increases the risk of marginal mucosal recession and adverse esthetic outcome Patient has high esthetic expectations
Complexity	High	Multiple staged procedures are required Technically demanding procedures
Risk of complications	High	Risk of complications is increased by the number of procedures and by their complexity
Loading protocol	Early	Loading within 12 weeks of implant placement following successful ridge augmentation procedures
SAC classification	Complex	

Tooth 21 was extracted (Figures 3 and 4) and loss of the facial bone wall was confirmed. Further evaluation of the site was deferred until after soft tissue healing had taken place. A bonded bridge was used as an interim replacement. The patient returned four weeks after extraction, and clinical and radiographic examination indicated a combined horizontal and vertical defect (Figures 5 to 7). The interproximal bony peaks were maintained; thus the prognosis for an acceptable esthetic result was favorable. The treatment plan – a staged approach, commencing with a ridge augmentation procedure and followed by implant placement six months later – was then confirmed.

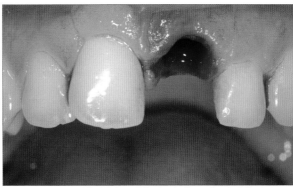

Figure 3.   Intra-oral facial view of the 21 site immediately following careful extraction of the tooth. Intraoperative assessment confirmed damage to the facial socket wall.

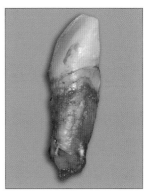

Figure 4.   The extracted tooth 21.

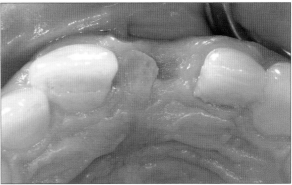

Figure 5.   Occlusal view of the 21 site after four weeks of healing. Horizontal resorption of the ridge was evident even at this early stage of healing.

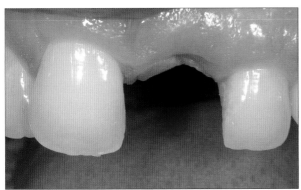

Figure 6.   Facial view of the healing 21 site four weeks after extraction. The bonded bridge was removed at this appointment to allow assessment of the site.

Figure 7.   Radiographic view of the 21 site four weeks after extraction, with the bonded provisional bridge in place. Clinical and radiological assessment at this time suggested a combined vertical and horizontal defect.

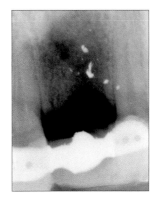

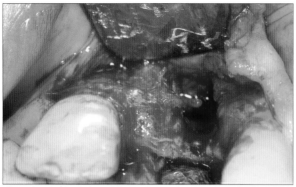

Figure 8.   Occlusal view of the healing socket following reflection of full-thickness mucoperiosteal flaps. Loss of horizontal bone dimension is evident.

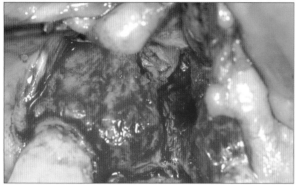

Figure 9.   Facial view of the healing site following flap reflection. Note the vertical loss of the facial bone wall of the healing extraction socket.

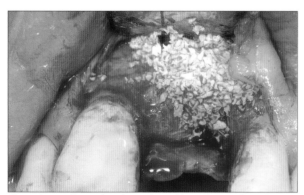

Figure 10.   A mixture of autologous bone chips and xenograft (bovine bone mineral) was used to fill the socket defect and to overlay the facial bone.

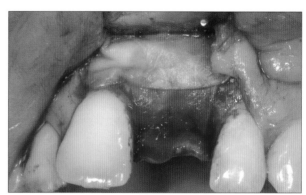

Figure 11.   The bone graft was covered with two layers of resorbable collagen membrane. Only one vertical releasing incision was used in this case.

Full-thickness flaps were raised with a small releasing incision on the distal aspect of tooth 11 (Figures 8 and 9). The defect was grafted with a mixture of autogenous bone (locally harvested) and deproteinized bovine bone mineral (BioOss, Geistlich Pharma AG, Wolhusen, Switzerland) (Figure 10). The facial bone was overlaid with the bone graft. Two layers of a resorbable membrane (BioGide, Geistlich Pharma AG, Wolhusen, Switzerland) were applied over the graft and surrounding native bone (Figure 11). After two weeks at suture removal, a bonded bridge was inserted as a provisional restoration.

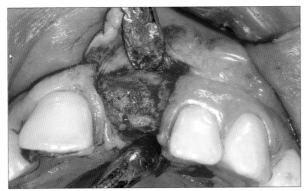

Figure 12.   Intraoperative occlusal view of the site six months later. Note the complete restitution of the dimensions of the ridge. The flap was designed so that the papillae and marginal tissues of the adjacent teeth were not reflected.

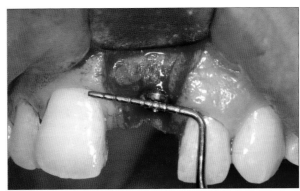

Figure 13.   Intra-operative facial view of the implant in position. The shoulder was located 2 mm apical to the gingival margin level of the adjacent teeth.

Six months later, the site was re-entered using a conservative flap design. A Straumann SLA implant (Straumann Implant System, Straumann AG, Basel, Switzerland) was carefully positioned with the shoulder located 2 mm apical to the gingival margin level of the adjacent teeth (Figures 12 to 14). The apico-coronal position of the implant shoulder was within the comfort zone, in accordance with the recommendations of the 2003 ITI Consensus Conference. The flaps were closed to facilitate submerged healing.

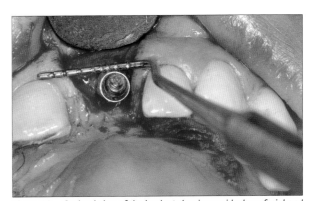

Figure 14.   Occlusal view of the implant showing an ideal oro-facial and mesio-distal position of the implant within the comfort zone, according to the recommendations of the 2003 ITI Consensus Conference. A submerged healing protocol was used during the integration phase.

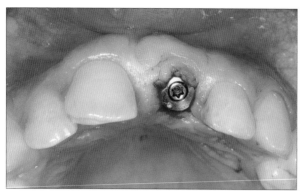

Figure 15.   After eight weeks of healing, the implant was uncovered with a minimal flap elevation. A beveled healing cap was inserted to start soft tissue conditioning.

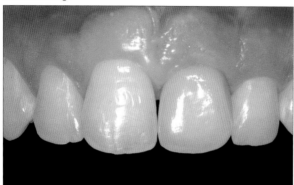

Figure 16.   Intra-oral facial view of the completed implant-supported restoration replacing 21.

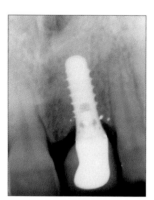

Figure 17.   Radiograph of the final case.

After a healing period of eight weeks, the shoulder of the implant was exposed with a minor flap elevation, and a beveled healing cap was applied (Figure 15). Restorative treatment was completed after five months of provisional loading (Figures 16 and 17).

In this case the surgical treatment consisted of four steps: extraction, reconstruction, implant placement, and implant uncovering. The overall surgical treatment of this case presents high esthetic risk, a high risk of complications, and high complexity of the involved procedures. This case should be considered *Complex*.

4.7 Implants for Restoration of Short Edentulous Spaces in Areas of High Esthetic Risk

D. Buser

Table 1 details the classification for clinical cases in the anterior maxilla with two to four adjacent missing teeth to be replaced by a prosthesis supported by two implants. It should be noted that none of the potential situations has a normative classification of *Straightforward*. These indications are all either *Advanced* or *Complex* due to several factors. One is that the inserted implants have to be positioned very precisely from a three-dimensional point of view. The concept of the *Comfort* and *Danger Zones* established by the ITI Consensus Conference in 2003 (Buser et al. 2004) needs to be applied. Surgical stents are routinely used in these clinical situations. Clinical experience has clearly shown that adjacent implants should be avoided whenever possible, since adjacent implants most often cause a reduced interimplant soft tissue height, which may lead to an impaired esthetic outcome (Tarnow et al. 2003). In addition, the bone width and/or height is often compromised when multiple adjacent teeth are missing or are planned for extraction. Bone augmentation, either simultaneous with implant placement or as a staged approach prior to implant placement, is usually required. In difficult cases, bone augmentation needs to be combined with adjunctive soft tissue grafts, either prior to, simultaneously with, or after implant placement. As a consequence, these clinical situations are demanding for the clinicians involved, since they require clinical experience for the selection of the appropriate treatment approach. The best sites for the implants need to be chosen in order to ensure optimal functional and esthetic outcomes. This decision must be based on a thorough esthetic risk assessment (Martin et al. 2007). In addition, an appropriately trained and skillful surgeon is needed to perform the necessary procedures with precision.

When the bone is deficient horizontally but the implant sites demonstrate favorable defect morphology, a simultaneous bone augmentation procedure (e.g., the GBR technique) is feasible at the time of implant placement. This is possible when the bone crest has sufficient oro-facial width and demonstrates a defect morphology of at least two bone walls. This situation is most often seen in early post-extraction sites. The need for adjunctive techniques increases the degree of difficulty of the treatment, resulting in a normative classification of *Advanced*.

If the site is deficient horizontally to a degree that bone augmentation is required prior to implant placement, the level of difficulty of the treatment increases significantly. This is usually necessary when the crest width measures 4 mm or less. Techniques for lateral bone augmentation may require combinations of autogenous bone grafts (block and/or particulate) or bone substitutes, tenting mechanisms for space maintenance, or barrier membranes (resorbable, non-resorbable and/or reinforced), depending upon the surgeon's preference. The level of difficulty is high, with a moderate risk of complications. The normative classification is *Complex* for this case type.

The normative classification of *Complex* also applies to clinical situations in which vertical bone deficiencies are present either at the implant site or at adjacent roots. These vertical deficiencies always cause compromised esthetic outcomes, and the level of difficulty is high.

Table 1. Surgical Classification of Cases in Short Edentulous Spaces in Areas of High Esthetic Risk.

Areas of High Esthetic Risk	Case Type: Short Edentulous Space					
Risk Assessment					Normative Classification	Notes/Adjunctive Procedures that may be required
Bone Volume	Anatomic Risk	Esthetic Risk	Complexity	Risk of Complications		
Defining Characteristics: Two implants and up to 4 teeth replaced						
Sufficient	Low	High	Moderate	Moderate	Advanced	Adjunctive soft tissue graft
Deficient horizontally, allowing simultaneous grafting	Low	High	Moderate	Moderate	Advanced	Adjunctive soft tissue graft Procedures for simultaneous horizontal bone augmentation In the anterior maxilla, the nasopalatine canal may increase the anatomic risk and influence implant position
Deficient horizontally, requiring prior grafting	Low	High	Moderate	Moderate	Complex	Adjunctive soft tissue graft Procedures for horizontal bone augmentation In the anterior maxilla, the nasopalatine canal may increase the anatomic risk and influence implant position
Deficient vertically and/or horizontally	High	High	High	High	Complex	Adjunctive soft tissue graft Risk to adjacent teeth Procedures for vertical and/or horizontal bone augmentation In the anterior maxilla, the nasopalatine canal may increase the anatomic risk and influence implant position

4.7.1 Clinical Case – Three Upper Anterior Teeth Requiring Extraction and Replacement with an Implant FDP

This is a case of a 28-year-old female patient who presented with a challenging situation in the anterior maxilla. The clinical status exhibited significant gingival recession associated with teeth 11, 21 and 22 (Figure 1). The periapical radiograph showed a vertical bone loss in this site (Figure 2). The patient was mainly disturbed by the gingival recession and the dark spaces between the three teeth, which were clearly visible when she smiled despite the medium smile line (Figure 3). To resolve the situation, it was planned to extract the three teeth and to insert two implants in positions 11 and 22 as abutments for a three-unit FDP. To achieve a satisfactory esthetic outcome, the main challenge was to regain bone height in the pontic area. Therefore, orthodontic extrusion of the three teeth was considered in order to gain as much soft tissue and bone height as possible prior to extraction of the teeth.

The following factors were considered in determining the SAC Classification for this case. The treatment plan required a combination of orthodontic treatment, tooth extraction, and implant placement, to be carried out in a staged approach. This would necessitate treatment to be completed over an extended period of time and with a high level of patient compliance. The patient's smoking habit was regarded as a risk for adverse soft tissue healing. Although the anatomic risk was low, there was a potential for the nasopalatine canal to influence the position of the 11 implant, which could further affect the esthetic result. Loss of ridge height in the 21 pontic region was identified as a significant esthetic risk factor. Even with orthodontic extrusion, bone augmentation to gain horizontal and vertical bone height at the time of implant placement was anticipated. For these reasons, the planned treatment had a high degree of complexity and an increased risk of adverse esthetic outcomes. The case was therefore classified as *Complex* (Table 2).

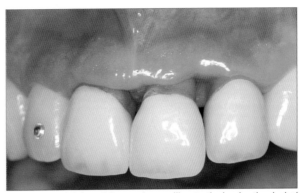

Figure 1.   Facial view of the anterior maxillary teeth, showing the gingival recession and loss of papillae.

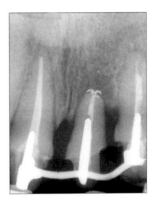

Figure 2.   A radiographic view of teeth 11, 21 and 22. Note the severe loss of bone height.

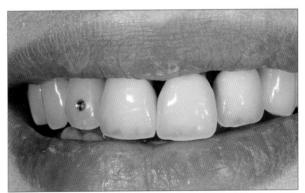

Figure 3.   This photograph illustrates the patient's lip line when she smiled. Dark spaces could be seen where the interdental papillae were missing.

Table 2. Surgical SAC Classification for the Case of Three Upper Anterior Teeth Requiring Extraction and Replacement with an Implant-Supported FDP.

General Factors	Assessment	Notes
Medical contraindications	None	
Smoking habit	< 10 cig/day	Patient was asked to stop smoking as soon as possible
Growth considerations	None	
Site Factors	**Assessment**	**Notes**
Bone volume	Insufficient	Horizontal and vertical deficiency
Anatomic risk	Low	The nasopalatine canal may interfere with ideal implant placement in the 11 site
Esthetic risk	High	Situation with multiple missing teeth, and pre-existing loss of the interdental papillae in a patient with a medium smile line Ridge height needs to be gained in the pontic region for optimum esthetics
Complexity	High	Combined horizontal and vertical augmentation required for an optimal result Adjunctive treatment in the form of orthodontic extrusion of the roots
Risk of complications	High	High risk of esthetic complications due to difficulty in achieving vertical augmentation
SAC Classification	Complex	

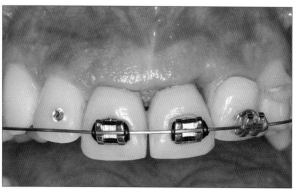

Figure 4.   Facial view of the maxillary anterior dentition following ortho-dontic treatment to extrude teeth 11, 21 and 22.

This demanding clinical situation required a comprehensive treatment in various steps. Initially, orthodontic treatment was used to extrude the teeth. The concept of forced eruption helped to regain some of the lost tissue height in this area (Figure 4).

At the next step, the three teeth were carefully extracted and the soft tissues were left to heal (Figure 5). After eight weeks, the soft tissues were sufficiently healed to allow the placement of two implants (Figure 6). To optimize a correct three-dimensional position of both implants, a surgical stent was used during surgery (Figure 7).

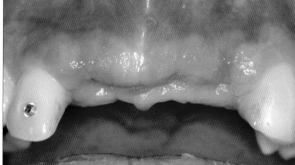

Figure 5.   Occlusal view of the ridge following extraction of 11, 21 and 22.

Figure 6.   Facial view of the ridge 8 weeks after extraction.

The localized bone defects were simultaneously augmented with autogenous bone and a bone filler with a low substitution rate (deproteinized bovine bone mineral). Special emphasis was placed on vertical augmentation in the pontic area (Figure 8).

Following application of a resorbable barrier membrane and primary wound closure, a healing period of 12 weeks was allowed to elapse before the implants were uncovered with a punch technique. The two implants were restored with a FDP.

The final restoration 18 months post implant placement demonstrated a pleasing result from an esthetic point of view (Figures 9 and 10). The black triangles were resolved between the prosthetic teeth by lengthening the contact regions. The radiograph at 18 months showed the successful vertical augmentation in the pontic area (Figure 11).

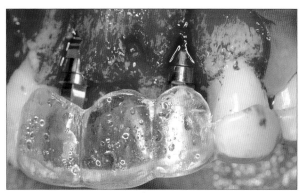

Figure 7. Facial view at the time of surgery. The implant sites were prepared with reference to a surgical guide to optimize the three-dimensional positioning of the implants. Note the dehiscences of the facial bone walls.

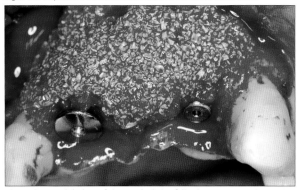

Figure 8. Facial view of the surgical site following augmentation with a bone graft.

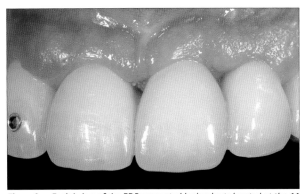

Figure 9. Facial view of the FDP supported by implants located at the 11 and 22 positions, 18 months after implant surgery.

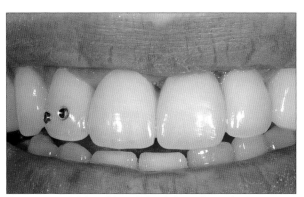

Figure 10. Facial view of the smile in relation to the new implant-supported FDP.

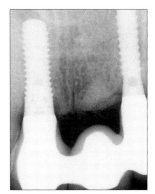

Figure 11. Radiographic appearance of the two implants at 18 months post-implant placement.

4.8 Implants for Prosthetic Replacement in Long Edentulous Spaces in Sites of High Esthetic Risk

S. Chen

In Table 1, the classifications for clinical situations in the anterior maxilla with more than two implants and more than three missing teeth are presented. It should be noted that all indications in this category are regarded as having normative classifications of *Advanced* or *Complex*. As described in the previous section, a high level of precision in prosthetic planning and surgical placement is required in order to achieve an optimal esthetic and functional result. Surgical stents are routinely used in these situations based on a thorough esthetic risk assessment (Martin et al. 2007) and diagnostic set-up. In these situations, adjacent implants often need to be considered. If so, sufficient space needs to be allowed between implants to minimize the loss of inter-implant crestal bone and to maintain the inter-implant soft tissue height (Tarnow et al. 2000). In addition, the bone width and/or height may often be compromised, requiring simultaneous or staged bone augmentation procedures. Where multiple teeth have been missing for some time, the resorption of the ridge may be significant. In difficult cases, bone augmentation needs to be combined with adjunctive soft tissue grafts, either prior to, simultaneous with, or after implant placement. In many instances, it is not possible to reconstruct the hard and soft tissues to pretreatment conditions. A flange is often incorporated into the final prosthesis for lip support, phonetics and esthetic outcomes. These factors need to be carefully assessed prior to commencement of treatment. As a consequence, these clinical situations are demanding for both the surgeon and the restorative dentist.

If the implant sites have sufficient bone volume, the placement of three or more implants in an area of high esthetic risk should be regarded as treatment of moderate complexity with a moderate risk of esthetic complications. Adjunctive soft tissue grafts are often required to improve the esthetic outcome. The normative classification is *Advanced* for this case type. When the bone is deficient horizontally, but the implant sites have favorable defect morphology, incorporating at least two intact bone walls, a simultaneous bone augmentation procedure may be undertaken at the time of implant placement. The normative classification for this process is also *Advanced*. It should be noted that if one or more adjacent implants are to be placed in these cases, the complexity of treatment and risk for esthetic complications may increase. The classification may need to be altered to *Complex* to reflect this elevated risk.

If the site is deficient horizontally to a degree that bone augmentation is required prior to implant placement, or if both a horizontal and a vertical ridge deficiency exists, techniques for lateral and/or vertical bone augmentation are required. Combinations of autogenous bone grafts (block and/or particulate) or bone substitutes, tenting mechanisms for space maintenance, barrier membranes (resorbable, non-resorbable and/or reinforced) and distraction osteogenesis may be considered. The level of difficulty is moderate to high, with a moderate to high risk of complications depending upon the treatment method selected. The normative classification is *Complex* for these case types.

Table 1. Surgical Classification of Cases in Long Edentulous Spaces in Areas of High Esthetic Risk.

Areas of High Esthetic Risk	Case Type: Long Span					
Risk Assessment					Normative Classification	Notes/Adjunctive Procedures that may be required
Bone Volume	Anatomic Risk	Esthetic Risk	Complexity	Risk of Complications		
Defining Characteristics: More than 2 implants, span of more than 3 teeth						
Sufficient	Low	High	Moderate	Moderate	Advanced	Adjunctive soft tissue graft Adjacent implants increase the complexity and risk of complications
Deficient horizontally, allowing simultaneous grafting	Low	High	Moderate	Moderate	Advanced	Adjunctive soft tissue graft Procedures for simultaneous horizontal bone augmentation The nasopalatine canal may increase the anatomic risk and influence implant position Adjacent implants increase the complexity and risk of complications
Deficient horizontally, requiring prior grafting	Moderate	High	Moderate	Moderate	Complex	Adjunctive soft tissue graft Procedures for horizontal bone augmentation The nasopalatine canal may increase the anatomic risk and influence implant position Adjacent implants increase the complexity and risk of complications
Deficient vertically and/or horizontally	High	High	High	High	Complex	Adjunctive soft tissue graft Risk to adjacent teeth Procedures for vertical and/or horizontal bone augmentation The nasopalatine canal may increase the anatomic risk and influence implant position Adjacent implants increase the complexity and risk of complications

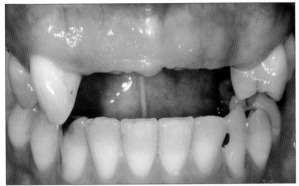

Figure 1.   Facial view of the patient's smile with the upper RDP in place.

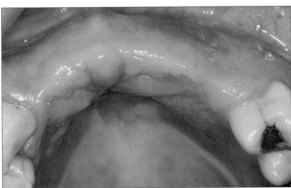

Figure 2.   Facial view of the edentulous ridge. Teeth 12, 11, 21, 22 and 23 were missing.

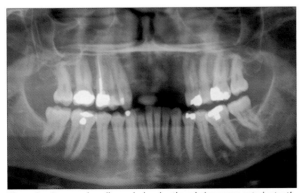

Figure 3.   Occlusal view of the edentulous ridge.

4.8.1   Clinical Case – Replacement of Five Missing Teeth in the Anterior Maxilla

A 50-year-old female patient presented with missing teeth 12, 11, 21, 22 and 23 in the anterior maxilla. The teeth had been lost many years previously following trauma. She had been wearing an upper removable dental prosthesis (RDP) and was interested in a fixed replacement for the missing teeth (Figure 1). Clinical examination revealed that she had a healthy, well-maintained dentition. The ridge showed good vertical height and minimal horizontal resorption (Figures 2 and 3). The lip line was low. A panoramic radiograph demonstrated good height of bone in the anterior maxilla (Figure 4). However, cone beam CT scans confirmed that marked horizontal resorption of the ridge had occurred, with the residual oro-facial dimension determined to be insufficient to allow implants to be placed (Figure 5).

The treatment plan was to carry out a bone augmentation procedure and to subsequently place three implants to support a five-unit FDP. There were no medical contraindications to treatment. However, the patient smoked cigarettes (fewer than 10 cigarettes per day). She was cautioned regarding the potential risk of surgical complications and risk to long-term success of the implant reconstruction as a result of her smoking habit. The need for horizontal augmentation of the ridge dictated a multi-staged surgical approach. A combination of cortico-cancellous autogenous block grafts and particulate deproteinized bovine bone mineral was proposed, with the retromolar mandibular region chosen as the donor site. The patient was advised of the risks and possible complications of this area as a donor site. The esthetic risk was determined to be moderate due to the favorable lip line. The patient was further advised that it was likely that a small flange would need to be incorporated in the final FDP to allow proper lip support, phonetics and esthetics.

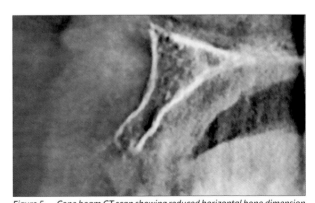

Figure 4.   Panoramic radiograph showing the missing upper anterior teeth, and ample vertical dimension of bone.

Figure 5.   Cone beam CT scan showing reduced horizontal bone dimension in the anterior maxilla

Table 2. Surgical SAC Classification for the Case of Five Missing Upper Anterior teeth Replaced with a FDP Supported by Three Implants.

General Factors	Assessment	Notes
Medical contraindications	None	
Smoking habit	< 10 ciga-rettes/day	
Growth considerations	None	
Site Factors	**Assessment**	**Notes**
Bone volume	Deficient horizontally	Staged bone augmentation procedure to increase horizontal bone dimensions required
Anatomic risk	Moderate	Secondary donor site increases the anatomic risk
Esthetic risk	Moderate	A flange may need to be incorporated in the FDP for lip support, tooth esthetics and phonetics The favorable lip line would allow the addition of a flange for ideal tooth and tissue esthetics
Complexity	High	Staged bone augmentation, secondary donor site, multiple surgical steps
Risk of complications	Moderate	Risk of complications from donor site Risk of complications at the graft site Incorporation of a flange in the FDP may create difficulties with access for maintenance and home-care
Loading protocol	Conventional	
SAC Classification	Complex	

For these reasons, the case was classified as *Complex* for the surgical phase of treatment (Table 2).

Treatment commenced with the bone augmentation procedure. Following flap reflection, the lack of sufficient horizontal width was confirmed (Figure 6). Two cortico-cancellous blocks of bone were harvested from the mandibular left retro-molar area and were grafted to the anterior maxillary ridge and stabilized with bone screws. Deproteinized bovine bone mineral (BioOss, Geistlich Pharma AG, Wolhusen, Switzerland) was used to fill the voids around the block grafts. A resorbable collagen membrane (BioGide, Geistlich Pharma AG, Wolhusen, Switzerland) was placed over the graft. Healing progressed uneventfully, and the site was re-opened after 6 months, revealing successful horizontal augmentation of the bony

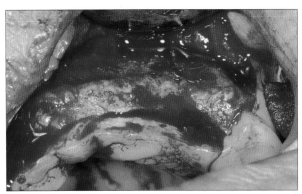

Figure 6. Surgical view of the ridge showing the facial concavity and lack of sufficient horizontal bone width.

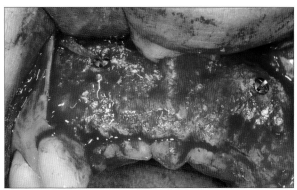

Figure 7. Surgical re-entry view six months following augmentation of the ridge, with a combination of autogenous cortical block grafts and deproteinized bovine bone mineral.

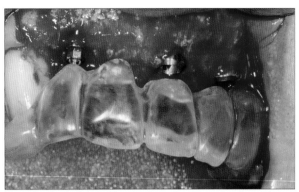

Figure 8.   Surgical view of three implants placed in conjunction with a surgical guide stent.

ridge (Figure 7). Three implants were placed using a surgical guide stent to achieve ideal implant position and axial orientation (Figure 8). A 10 mm narrow-neck implant (Straumann Narrow-neck implant, Straumann AG, Basel, Switzerland) was placed in the 12 site. Two 10 mm-long implants (Straumann RN Standard Plus implants, Straumann AG, Basel, Switzerland) were placed in the 21 and 23 sites. This plan avoided the placement of adjacent implants. The implants successfully integrated and were restored with a five-unit porcelain-fused-to-metal (PFM) FDP retained by transverse screws (Figures 9 to 11).

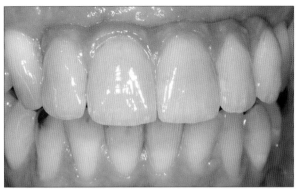

Figure 9.   Facial view of the completed implant-supported FDP. A flange in pink porcelain was constructed for lip support and phonetics.

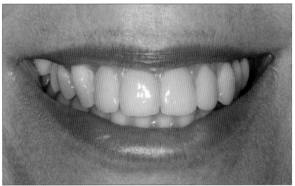

Figure 10.   Extra-oral facial view showing the patient's smile with completed FDP in place one year after loading.

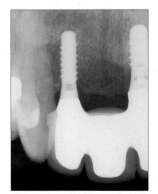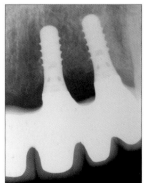

Figures 11a and 11b.   Periapical radiographs of the completed case one year after delivery of the FDP.

4.9 Implants for Restoration of Full Arches in Areas of High Esthetic Risk

L. Cordaro

The edentulous maxilla should be regarded as a region of high esthetic risk due to the need to replace the maxillary anterior teeth and to restore proper lip support. There are different treatment options for management of the edentulous upper jaw. The surgeon should conduct detailed discussions and planning with both the patient and the restorative dentist to arrive at an appropriate treatment plan. The decision of the type of prosthesis depends on various factors: the volume of residual bone, the interocclusal space, the intermaxillary relationship, lip support, phonetics and economic considerations. Once the decision for a fixed or a removable prosthesis has been made, a number of variables need to be considered to define the normative classification for a particular case.

Table 1 describes the normative classification for the surgical implant treatment of the fully edentulous upper arch. Usually an overdenture in the maxilla is retained by four implants, but some clinicians may plan the insertion of a larger number (from six to eight), especially in cases with poor bone quality and quantity. Although the following discussion refers to a treatment plan consisting of four implants to retain an overdenture, similar considerations apply to cases in which overdentures are to be retained by more than four implants. It should be noted that the normative classification may need to be modified to reflect the increased surgical complexity involved in placing additional implants and for cases in which bone quality and quantity are sub-optimal.

If an overdenture retained by four implants is planned and the bone volume is sufficient, the anatomical risk, complexity of the procedure, and risk of complications are regarded as low. Although the esthetic risk is high, the type of prosthesis allows many of the esthetic problems to be resolved. The SAC Classification for these cases is *Straightforward*. The inter-maxillary relationship should be considered with great caution, since the space occupied by a retentive bar and the attachments may interfere with the correct positioning of the teeth on the final prosthesis. Lack of sufficient vertical space will alter the normative classification.

In similar cases showing horizontal ridge deficiencies that may be corrected at the time of implant placement, the

normative classification is *Advanced*. At the time of implant placement, augmentation procedures may be used to correct fenestrations or dehiscence defects. The anatomical risk is regarded as low; however, the risk of complications and complexity of the procedure are moderately high.

If the alveolar ridge is deficient horizontally and a bony reconstruction is to be carried out as a separate surgical step some months before implant insertion, the normative classification is *Complex*. Usually these cases are treated with autogenous block grafts harvested from intra-oral or extra-oral sites. In some instances the alveolar width may be augmented with GBR techniques that involve the use of barrier membranes and autogenous chips and/or xenografts or allografts. When a harvesting procedure is needed, the added morbidity associated with a second surgical site needs to be considered. For these reasons, the complexity and the risk of complications of these procedures are elevated to a high degree.

Similarly, if an overdenture is planned in cases in which reduced height of the residual ridge precludes implant placement, the normative classification is also *Complex*. In these cases a staged approach is recommended, involving vertical bone augmentation followed by implant placement after maturation of the grafts. Bone augmentation is usually achieved in an occlusal direction with bone blocks. These procedures are very demanding from a technical point of view. In some cases the vertical reconstruction may be achieved with elevation of the floor of the maxillary sinus or the floor of the nose. Surgery involving the floor of the nose or the sinus is considered complex because the anatomical risk is high and there is a high risk of complications. If a bone harvesting procedure is needed, the complexity of the treatment is further increased due to the morbidity associated with the donor site.

When addressing the normative classification of the surgical treatment of an edentulous maxilla that is to be rehabilitated with a fixed prosthesis, some preliminary considerations need to be made. From a prosthetic point of view, there are two factors which may influence the surgical treatment plan and consequently affect the normative classification.

Table 1. Surgical Classification of Full-arch Cases in Areas of High Esthetic Risk.

Areas of High Esthetic Risk	Case Type: Full Arch – Maxilla					
Risk Assessment					**Normative Classification**	**Notes/Adjunctive Procedures that may be required**
Bone Volume	**Anatomic Risk**	**Esthetic Risk**	**Complexity**	**Risk of Complications**		
Defining Characteristics: 4 implants, overdenture						
Sufficient	Low	High	Low	Low	Straight-forward	Relative alignment of implants Intraocclusal distance
Deficient horizontally, but allowing simultaneous augmentation	Low	High	Moderate	Moderate	Advanced	Relative alignment of implants Procedures for simultaneous horizontal bone augmentation
Deficient horizontally, requiring prior bone augmentation	Low	High	High	High	Complex	Relative alignment of implants Procedures for prior horizontal bone augmentation
Deficient vertically and/or horizontally, requiring prior bone augmentation	High	High	High	High	Complex	Relative alignment of implants Maxillary sinus involvement Procedures for prior vertical and horizontal bone augmentation
Defining Characteristics: 5 or more implants, fixed hybrid bridge						
Sufficient	Low	High	Moderate	Low	Advanced	Relative alignment of implants
Deficient horizontally, but allowing simultaneous augmentation	Moderate	High	High	High	Complex	Maxillary sinus involvement Procedures for simultaneous horizontal bone augmentation Relative alignment of implants
Deficient horizontally, requiring prior bone augmentation	Moderate	High	High	High	Complex	Maxillary sinus involvement Procedures for prior horizontal bone augmentation Relative alignment of implants
Deficient vertically and/or horizontally, requiring prior bone augmentation	High	High	High	High	Complex	Maxillary sinus involvement Procedures for prior vertical and/or horizontal bone augmentation Relative alignment of implants
Defining Characteristics: 6 or more implants, immediate loading						
Sufficient	Low	High	High	High	Complex	Relative alignment of implants

First, if there is sufficient hard and soft tissue volume to allow the placement of a FDP that does not require a flange to replace missing soft tissue, precise three-dimensional placement of the implants is required. This mandates implant placements where the implant shoulders are coincident with the cervical emergence of the prosthetic teeth. However, where a flange is necessary for esthetics and/or phonetics, the need for precise positioning of the implants is less demanding. In this case, a hybrid prosthesis may be used. This type of prosthesis replaces not only the teeth but also part of the bone and soft tissues that were lost together with the teeth.

Second, if five or more implants are needed to support a fixed or hybrid restoration and an adequate volume of bone is present, the procedure is considered *Advanced*. The anatomical risk and the risk of complications are low, but the procedure has a moderate complexity. The esthetic risk is likely to be high, as the esthetic zone is involved.

In all other anatomical situations of the upper jaw for which a full-arch fixed rehabilitation is planned, the surgical part of the treatment must be considered *Complex* and a high degree of expertise is needed. This is true for cases in which the horizontal ridge deficiency can be corrected at the time of implant placement as well as for those requiring a staged procedure. In these cases the risk of complications, the complexity of the procedure, and the esthetic risk are high and are associated with a moderate anatomical risk. If a simultaneous augmentation procedure can be carried out, GBR procedures are used with particulate grafting materials and barrier membranes. When a staged approach is indicated, block grafts are usually used.

If a vertical bony deficiency is present and the prosthetic treatment plan calls for a vertical augmentation in an apical direction (i.e. elevation of the floor of the maxillary sinus), the complexity and risk of the procedure are high. Some cases may be treated with alloplasts or xenografts, thus eliminating the need for a second surgical access related to bone harvesting. If the treatment plan requires vertical augmentation in the occlusal direction, a very demanding grafting procedure has to be carried out after careful evaluation of the amount of vertical augmentation needed. In these cases not only does the surgical procedure itself present a high risk of complications, but the entire healing phase has to be carefully monitored because of the possible interference caused by the interim removable prosthesis.

In some cases the maxillary atrophy is so advanced and the intermaxillary relationship is so unfavorable that a simultaneous Le Fort I osteotomy and extensive grafting procedures are planned. In this case the procedure allows

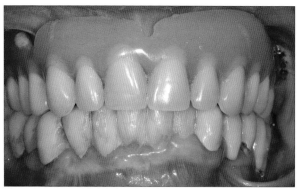

Figure 1. Intraoral facial view of the full upper denture opposing a natural lower dentition.

for simultaneous three-dimensional repositioning of the upper jaw in a correct position, and augmentation of the residual alveolar ridge. This procedure is defined as *Complex*. It is carried out as an inpatient procedure under general anesthesia, and should be performed by experienced oral and maxillofacial surgeons.

Immediate loading procedures are considered *Complex*. From a surgical point of view, when prosthetic loading with a complete arch FDP is planned, some additional difficulties are involved in the surgical phase, such as achievement of high primary stability of each implant and very accurate three-dimensional positioning of the implants compatible with the previously planned provisional restoration. In some teams it may also be the case that the provisional prosthetic treatment is performed by the surgeon himself, who needs to have prosthetic expertise.

4.9.1   Clinical Case – An Implant-Supported FDP in an Edentulous Maxilla

A 65-year-old woman with a removable prosthesis in the upper jaw and a failing fixed rehabilitation in the lower jaw (Figure 1) asked for a fixed rehabilitation in the upper jaw. The patient had poor oral hygiene. A panoramic radi-

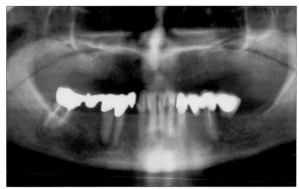

Figure 2.   Pre-treatment panoramic radiograph of the patient's dentition.

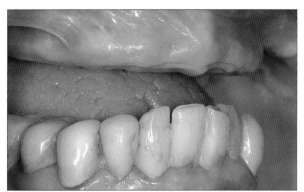

Figure 3.   Oblique anterior view of the edentulous maxilla showing the relationship of the upper ridge to the lower anterior teeth.

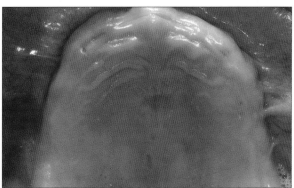

Figure 4.   Occlusal view of the edentulous maxilla.

ograph showed adequate bone height anterior to the maxillary sinuses (Figure 2). This was discussed with the patient, who refused augmentation procedures involving the floor of the sinus. The edentulous ridge was well formed, with a favorable anterior relationship between the ridge and lower teeth (Figures 3 and 4).

Following completion of an initial hygienic phase, a diagnostic set-up was prepared. This demonstrated the possibility of a complete arch FDP supported by six implants placed anteriorly to the maxillary sinuses. The planned implant positions were the central incisor, canine, and second premolar sites bilaterally to support a 12-unit FDP with two-unit distal cantilevers. The patient had a high lip line, displaying 2 mm of the soft tissues in the diagnostic setup. It was determined that sufficient lip support could be achieved without the need for a flange. In the mandible it was decided to extract the right second molar due to recurrent caries and to provide the patient with a tooth-supported FDP from second premolar to second premolar. Two implants would be needed to replace the first molars with two implant-supported single crowns. With this plan, the patient's rehabilitation would include 12 units in the upper and lower jaws.

Several factors were considered when determining the SAC Classification for this case. The anatomic risk was low since it was decided not to operate in the area of maxillary sinus. However, the proximity of the nasopalatine canal would need to be assessed at the time of surgery, as this could influence the position of the implants in the central incisor sites. The complexity of the surgical procedure was determined to be moderate due to the number of implants to be placed and the care required to avoid excessive divergence of the implants. The risk of complications was regarded as low; however, care would be required in placement of the most distal implants, in order to avoid the sinuses. The esthetic risk was high, and very precise positioning of the implants would be required. An early loading protocol was planned. These factors contributed to an SAC Classification of *Advanced* for this case (Table 2).

Table 2. Surgical SAC Classification for the Case of an Implant-Supported FDP in an Edentulous Maxilla Supported by 6 Implants.

General Factors	Assessment	Notes
Medical contraindications	None	
Smoking habit	None	
Growth considerations	None	
Site Factors	**Assessment**	**Notes**
Bone volume	Adequate in the anterior and premolar regions of the maxilla Vertical deficiency in the molar area	Sufficient bone volume was anticipated in the maxillary anterior and premolar sites without the need for adjunctive bone augmentation.
Anatomic risk	Low	The nasopalatine canal could affect the position of implants planned in the central incisor sites
Esthetic risk	High	On full smile, 2 mm of soft tissue would be visible.
Complexity	Moderate	Care would be required to prevent implants being placed with excessive divergence The most distal implants would be close to the maxillary sinuses
Risk of complications	Low	Care would be required during the initial healing phase to avoid premature loading of the implants
Loading protocol	Early	Loading between 6 and 12 weeks following implant placement
SAC Classification	Advanced	

The diagnostic wax-up was duplicated to allow fabrication of a surgical stent. Surgical access was achieved with a crestal incision from molar site to the contralateral molar site. Two distal vertical releasing incisions allowed for adequate flap reflection and visualization of the ridge. Six SLA implants, 4.1 mm in diameter and 10 and 12 mm in length (Straumann Implant System, Straumann AG, Basel, Switzerland) were inserted in the planned positions using the surgical stent for guidance. Flaps were closed to allow transmucosal healing (Figures 5 and 6). During the healing phase the old removable prosthesis was used by the patient, but it was relined with soft acrylic and relieved at the implant sites to avoid premature indirect loading of the implants. The definitive prosthetic phase commenced

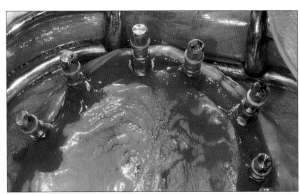

Figure 5.   Occlusal view of the maxilla following installation of six implants.

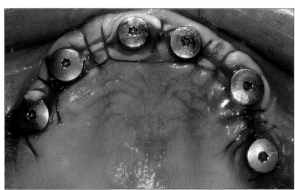

Figure 6.   After attachment of healing caps, the flaps were adapted to the healing caps and closed with interrupted sutures. A transmucosal healing protocol was followed.

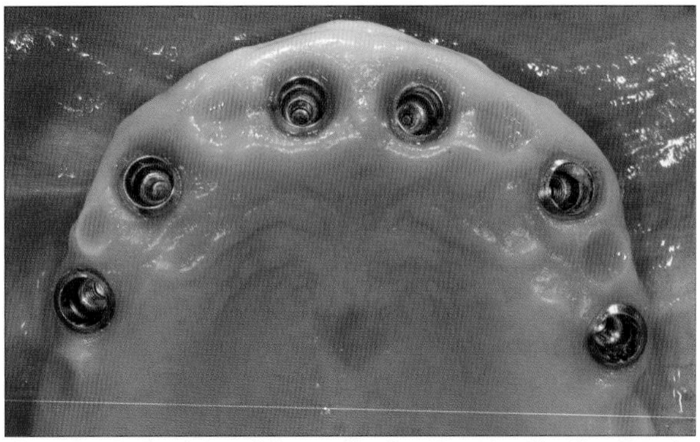

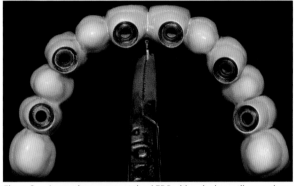

Figure 7.   Occlusal view of the maxilla after 10 weeks of healing. Note the healthy mucosa at the implant sites with healing caps removed, and the initial soft tissue conditioning obtained with the provisional restoration.

8 weeks after surgery, and included the use of a full-arch provisional fixed restoration for 4 weeks to allow soft tissue conditioning before definitive impressions could be taken (Figure 7). The patient was rehabilitated with a one-piece screw-retained FDP with one cantilever unit per side. Two implants were placed to replace the first molars with two implant-supported single crowns. For hygienic reasons it was decided to prepare the mandibular abutment teeth so as to leave the supra-gingival crown margins (Figures 8 to 10).

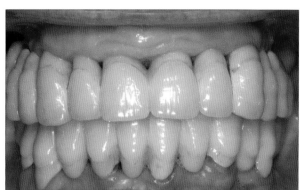

Figure 8.   A one-piece, screw-retained FDP with a single cantilever unit per side was fabricated to restore this case. In this case a Procera Implant Bridge (Nobel Biocare AG, Gothenburg, Sweden) made of porcelain fused to titanium was directly connected to the implants.

Figure 9.   Intra-oral facial view of the final implant-supported FDP in the maxilla and a tooth-supported FDP from second premolar to second premolar in the lower jaw. Two implants were used to replace the mandibular first molars with implant-supported crowns.

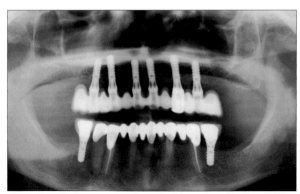

Figure 10.   Final panoramic radiograph of the patient after the rehabilitation.

4.10 Implants in Extraction Sockets (Type 1 Placement) of Single-Rooted Teeth

S. Chen

As extraction sockets present specific anatomical risks and treatment complexities, a separate classification has been proposed for single- and multi-rooted tooth sites. Implants in extraction sockets should therefore be considered as a specific modifying factor, which may alter the normative classification for a particular clinical indication.

Table 1 shows the classifications for implants placed in extraction sockets of single-rooted teeth. Following placement, most implants in extraction sockets present with a peri-implant defect. The decision to place a graft is usually based upon the dimensions of the marginal defect in a horizontal plane and/or loss of one or more socket walls. Although spontaneous regeneration of bone may be anticipated if the horizontal dimension is 2 mm or less (Paolantonio et al. 2001), this is accompanied by horizontal resorption of the facial bone wall (Botticelli et al. 2004). In esthetic sites, grafting of defects with allografts or xenografts with low substitution rates may be considered to reduce the horizontal resorption (Chen et al. 2007). If the horizontal dimension of the marginal defect is greater than 2 mm, a simultaneous augmentation procedure should be considered. If one or more socket walls is damaged or missing, simultaneous augmentation procedures should be undertaken using combinations of bone grafts and bone substitutes, and barrier membranes.

The normative classification for implants placed into the sockets of maxillary incisors and canines is *Complex* due to the potential for esthetic complications if there is recession of the facial marginal mucosa. The risk of marginal mucosal recession may be moderate or high depending upon the condition of the facial socket wall and tissue biotype. If the facial socket wall is damaged or lost and/or the tissues are thin, the risks of recession and esthetic complications are elevated. If the esthetic risk is high, then an early placement protocol (Type 2 placement) is recommended. This approach allows soft tissue healing and resolution of infection to take place after tooth extraction. There is an increase in the volume of mucosa which facilitates surgical flap management and/or primary wound closure if required. The osteotomy needs to be carefully performed to ensure that the implant achieves adequate initial stability and correct axial orientation. In maxillary incisor and canine sockets, this is achieved by preparing the osteotomy into the palatal wall of the socket. The palatal bone wall is also flared in the coronal third of the socket to reduce the risk of the implant deflecting towards the facial side during installation. Adjunctive augmentation procedures may be required to promote regeneration of bone in the defect adjacent to the implant. The procedure has a moderate degree of complexity. If one or more socket walls are damaged or missing, a simultaneous bone augmentation procedure is indicated. In many cases, simultaneous soft tissue grafting procedures should be considered to increase the volume of soft tissue for a submerged healing protocol and/or for improving the soft tissue form for optimum esthetic outcomes. This elevates the degree of complexity of the treatment. The anatomic risk is generally regarded as low in these sites.

Mandibular premolars usually present as single-rooted teeth. The socket dimensions are similar to the dimensions of standard cylindrical or tapered implants offered by most implant systems, resulting in relatively small marginal defects. These sites usually have a low esthetic risk. If the socket walls are intact and the mental nerve and foramen are not in proximity, the normative classification is *Straightforward*. If, however, one or more socket walls are damaged, simultaneous bone augmentation procedures need to be performed, thereby raising the normative classification to *Advanced*. In mandibular premolar sites that are in close proximity to the mental foramen, the anatomical risks are elevated and hence the normative classification should be considered *Advanced*, whether bone augmentation procedures are required or not.

In the mandibular anterior region, the normative classification for implants placed into extraction sockets is *Advanced*. The facial/lingual walls are often thin, which increases the complexity of the surgical management. Mandibular incisor sites have reduced socket dimensions and often present with an oro-facial narrowing of the alveolar bone at the apex of the roots. This elevates the risk of perforation of the lingual cortex and subsequently the risk of complications arising from such a perforation. Whenever one or more socket walls have been damaged, a simultaneous bone augmentation procedure is required.

Table 1. Surgical Classification of Implants in Extraction Sockets (Type 1 Placement) of Single-Rooted Teeth.

Socket Morphology: Single Root						
Risk Assessment					**Normative Classification**	**Notes/Adjunctive Procedures that may be required**
Bone Volume	**Anatomic Risk**	**Esthetic Risk**	**Complexity**	**Risk of Complications**		
Tooth Site: Maxillary incisors and canines						
Sufficient, with intact bone walls	Low	High	Moderate	High	Complex	Procedures for simultaneous soft tissue grafting Procedures for simultaneous bone augmentation
Damage to one or more socket walls	Low	High	Moderate	High	Complex	Procedures for simultaneous soft tissue grafting Procedures for simultaneous bone augmentation
Tooth Site: Mandibular premolars						
Sufficient, with intact bone walls	Low	Low	Low	Low	Straightfor-ward	None
Damage to one or more socket walls	Low	Low	Moderate	Moderate	Advanced	Procedures for simultaneous bone augmentation
Tooth Site: Mandibular premolar, adjacent to mental foramen						
Sufficient, with intact bone walls	Moderate	Low	Moderate	Moderate	Advanced	Risk of mental nerve involvement
Damage to one or more socket walls	Moderate	Low	Moderate	Moderate	Advanced	Procedures for simultaneous bone augmentation Risk of Mental nerve involvement
Tooth Site: Mandibular incisors and canines						
Sufficient, with intact bone walls	Moderate	Low	Moderate	Moderate	Advanced	Lingual cortex perforation
Damage to one or more socket walls	Moderate	Low	Moderate	Moderate	Advanced	Lingual cortex perforation Procedures for simultaneous bone augmentation

4.10.1 Clinical Case – Replacement of a Maxillary Central Incisor with an Implant Placed at the Time of Extraction

A 36-year-old female patient presented with a failing upper left central incisor (tooth 21) with a discharging sinus at the mucogingival junction (Figure 1). The tooth had been endodontically treated and restored with a post-retained crown following trauma (Figure 2). The patient reported a history of recurrent infection and swelling of the gingiva. Although apical surgery that had been carried out two years previously was initially successful, the swelling and discharging sinus recurred a year later. Clinical examination confirmed an otherwise healthy dentition. The 21 had normal probing pocket depths of 2 to 3 mm. The patient's request was for a fixed replacement of this tooth. Her esthetic expectations were high due to the high lip line at full smile. The treatment plan was to extract the 21, and if possible, undertake simultaneous implant placement.

Although the probing pockets around the tooth were within normal limits, the history of recurrent infection and swelling and previous apical surgery suggested that there was damage to the facial bone wall. Thus implant placement at the time of extraction would require a simultaneous bone augmentation procedure. Bone volume apical to the area of infection appeared sufficient for initial implant stability. Although the anatomic risk was regarded as low, there was a possibility that the periapical area of bone loss communicated with the nasopalatine canal. The thick biotype and excess gingival height in relation to the adjacent central incisor were favorable clinical conditions for immediate (Type 1) implant placement. However, the condition of the facial bone wall increased the risk of marginal tissue recession. Given the high esthetic demands, the esthetic risk was determined to be high. The need for adjunctive bone augmentation increased the level of complexity of the treatment. Apart from the esthetic risk, the risk for other complications was low. The SAC Classification for this case was *Complex* (Table 2).

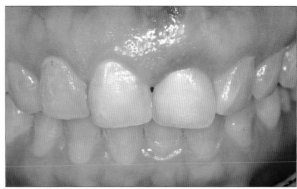

Figure 1.   Intraoral facial view of the upper left central incisor (tooth 21) with a discharging sinus.

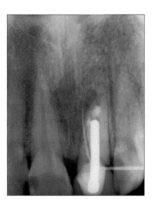

Figure 2.   Periapical radiograph of the upper left central incisor with a gutta percha point used to trace the sinus tract. A periapical radiolucency was evident on the mesial aspect of the root.

Table 2. Surgical SAC Classification for Replacement of a Maxillary Central Incisor with an Immediate (Type 1) Implant.

General Factors	Assessment	Notes
Medical contraindications	None	
Smoking habit	None	
Growth considerations	None	
Site Factors	**Assessment**	**Notes**
Bone volume	Adequate bone volume apical to the tooth The extent of damage to the facial bone wall could not be determined	Adjunctive hard tissue augmentation procedures required
Anatomic risk	Low	Proximity of the nasopalatine canal may affect the position of the implant
Esthetic risk	High	High lip line on full smile High patient esthetic demands Risk of marginal mucosal recession judged to be high due to damage of the facial bone wall. Thick tissue biotype and excess soft tissue height were favorable factors.
Complexity	High	Simultaneous bone augmentation in an area of high esthetic risk
Risk of complications	Low	Risk of failing to gain ideal initial stability Risk of a communication with the nasopalatine canal
SAC Classification	Complex	

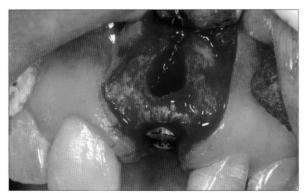

Figure 3.   Intraoperative view of the implant in place. Note the large fenestration of the facial bone wall and the intact bridge of bone at the crest.

After extraction of the 21, a large fenestration defect was evident (Figure 3). However, an intact bridge of bone of moderate thickness remained at the crest of the facial bone wall. Following implant installation (10 mm RN SP SLA implant; Straumann Implant System, Straumann AG, Basel, Switzerland), the resultant fenestration was grafted with deproteinized bovine bone mineral (BioOss, Geistlich Pharma AG, Wolhusen, Switzerland) and covered with a resorbable collagen membrane. The flap was sutured to facilitate semi-submerged healing (Figure 4). Healing progressed without incident (Figure 5). After 12 weeks, the implant was restored with a PFM crown. The clinical and radiographic conditions were stable two years following surgery, with a pleasing esthetic outcome (Figures 6 to 8).

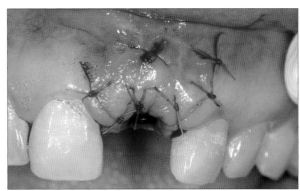

Figure 4.   Facial view of the surgical site following implant insertion, grafting of the defect, application of a resorbable barrier membrane, and flap closure. The healing cap was partially submerged.

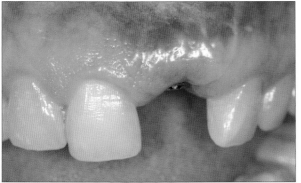

Figure 5.   After three months, the peri-implant mucosa was healthy.

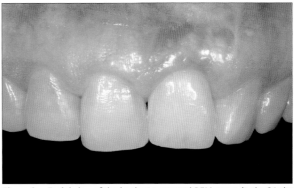

Figure 6.   Facial view of the implant-supported PFM crown in the 21 site two years following surgical placement.

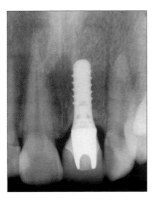

Figure 7.   Periapical radiograph of the 21 implant two years after surgery.

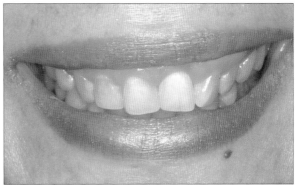

Figure 8.   The patient's smile, showing the 21 implant restoration two years after surgery.

4.11 Implants in Extraction Sockets (Type 1 Placement) of Multi-Rooted Teeth

S. Chen

The classifications for implants in multi-rooted extraction sockets are presented in Table 1. The morphology of multi-rooted sockets presents unique challenges for achieving an optimal implant position and initial implant stability.

Depending upon the morphology of the roots and height of the root trunk, there is often a thin inter-radicular septum between the facial and palatal sockets of maxillary premolars. Implants should ideally be placed in the oro-facial mid-point of the socket for proper three-dimensional positioning (Fugazzotto 2002). Initial stability is achieved by contact of the implant with the mesial and distal bone walls. The horizontal defect between the implants and facial and palatal bone walls may often be greater than 2 mm; therefore, simultaneous bone augmentation procedures are usually required. Immediate placement of implants in maxillary premolar sockets may be complicated by perforation of the facial wall at the infrazygomatic fossa, where a prominent concavity may be present. The maxillary sinus may extend anteriorly to involve the roots of these teeth. In the presence of damage to one or more socket walls, simultaneous bone augmentation procedures need to be carried out. For these reasons, the normative classification for implants placed into maxillary premolar extraction sites is *Advanced*.

In maxillary molar sites, three distinct root sockets are usually present. When there is sufficient bone height between the root apices and the floor of the maxillary sinus, initial implant stability is obtained by anchoring the implant in this apical bone. Implants should be placed in the oro-facial and mesio-distal midpoint of the sockets (Schwartz-Arad and Samet 1999). Placement of implants into the individual root sockets should be avoided, as this usually results in a poor restorative position of the implant. The anatomical and esthetic risks are regarded as low. The treatment is moderately complex and careful site preparation is required to achieve initial stability. Peri-implant defects may vary in size depending upon the diameter of the implant used. However, simultaneous bone augmentation procedures are generally required for implants placed into maxillary molar sockets. The normative classification is *Advanced*.

For cases in which the floor of the maxillary sinus is in close proximity to the root apices, there is usually insufficient apical bone to provide initial stability. In most cases, elevation of the sinus membrane and grafting of the sinus floor with a bone graft or substitute is required. This may be achieved using variations of the osteotome technique (Summers 1994, Fugazzotto 2006) or via a lateral window approach (Tatum 1986). Due to the presence of the root sockets, the sinus floor is irregular, which increases the risk of perforation of the sinus membrane during sinus floor grafting procedures. These cases are regarded as *Complex*, with a moderate level of risk of complications, and should be performed by experienced surgeons with a high level of skill.

In mandibular molar sites with adequate bone volume between the root apices and the mandibular canal, implant installation into the extraction sockets may be considered. Implants wider in diameter than standard implants are usually selected, and should be placed into the mesio-distal and oro-facial mid-points of the socket. Implant stability is achieved by contact with the facial and oral socket walls, and engagement of bone in the inter-radicular septum (if present) and the apical bone. Placement of implants into either the mesial or distal sockets may be considered, but only if there are restorative indications for this approach. The placement of two implants into the mesial and distal sockets should generally be avoided. The anatomical risk is regarded as low. The normative classification is *Advanced*.

If there is limited bone height between the base of the socket and the mandibular canal, the risk of damage to the Inferior Alveolar Nerve is high. The anatomical risk, risk of complications, and complexity are high. Placement of implants into mandibular molar sockets when there is limited bone height, or where there is damage to one or more of the socket walls, leads to a normative classification of *Complex*.

Table 1. Surgical Classification of Implants in Extraction Sockets (Type 1 Placement) of Multi-Rooted Teeth.

Socket Morphology: Multiple Roots						
Risk Assessment					**Normative Classification**	**Notes/Adjunctive Procedures that may be required**
Bone Volume	**Anatomic Risk**	**Esthetic Risk**	**Complexity**	**Risk of Complications**		
Tooth Site: Maxillary premolars						
Sufficient	Low	High	Moderate	Moderate	Advanced	Risk of perforating facial cortical bone Procedures for simultaneous soft tissue grafting Procedures for simultaneous bone augmentation
Damage to one or more socket walls	Low	High	Moderate	Moderate	Advanced	Risk of perforating facial cortical bone Procedures for simultaneous soft tissue grafting Procedures for simultaneous bone augmentation
Tooth Site: Maxillary molars						
Sufficient	Low	Low	Moderate	Moderate	Advanced	Procedures for simultaneous bone augmentation
Deficient vertically	Moderate	Low	High	High	Complex	Procedures for simultaneous sinus floor augmentation
Damage to one or more sockets walls with or without vertical deficiency	Moderate	Low	High	High	Complex	Procedures for simultaneous bone augmentation Procedures for simultaneous sinus floor augmentation
Tooth Site: Mandibular molars						
Sufficient	Low	Low	Moderate	Moderate	Advanced	Procedures for simultaneous bone augmentation
Deficient vertically	High	Low	High	High	Complex	Inferior dental nerve involvement Procedures for simultaneous bone augmentation
Damage to one or more socket walls with or without vertical deficiency	High	Low	High	High	Complex	Inferior dental nerve involvement Procedures for simultaneous bone augmentation

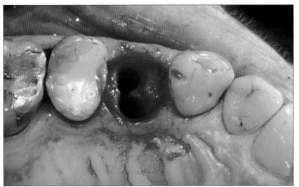

Figure 1.   Occlusal view of the upper right first premolar. A stainless steel band was placed around the tooth to support an interim restoration.

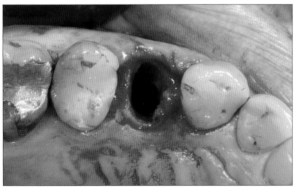

Figure 2.   Occlusal view of the site following extraction of the tooth. Note the two distinct sockets and the "kidney-shaped" coronal portion of the socket.

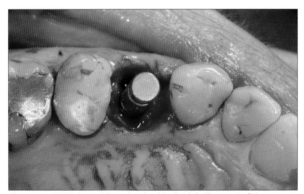

Figure 3.   Occlusal view of the site following preparation of the socket.

4.11.1 Clinical Case – Replacement of a Maxillary First Premolar with an Implant Placed at the Time of Extraction

A 55-year-old female patient presented with a subgingival fracture of the upper right first premolar (Figure 1). The patient requested a fixed replacement for this tooth. She was a healthy non-smoker with realistic esthetic expectations. Radiographic examination showed the presence of two distinct roots. The treatment plan was to extract the tooth and to place an implant into the extraction socket. The patient was willing to forgo wearing an interim removable prosthesis during the healing phase.

After administration of local anesthesia, sulcular incisions were made on the facial and palatal surfaces of the tooth. Using a combination of periotomes and fine luxators, the tooth was carefully extracted (Figure 2). Bone sounding was performed to determine the external contours of the facial and palatal bone walls. The osteotomy was then prepared into the oro-facial midpoint of the socket, with care taken to direct the preparation slightly to the palatal aspect to avoid perforating the facial bone (Figures 3 and 4). An implant with an endosseous length of 10 mm and an SLA surface (Straumann RN SP implant, Straumann AG, Basel, Switzerland) was then inserted into the osteotomy (Figure 5). A healing cap was then attached to the implant. The facial and palatal mucosa was then adapted

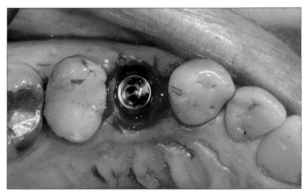

Figure 4.   Guide in position, showing ideal axial alignment of the osteotomy preparation.

Figure 5.   A RN Straumann implant in place. The small marginal gaps on the facial and oral sides of the implant shoulder were grafted with deproteinized bovine bone mineral.

Table 2. Surgical SAC Classification for Replacement of a Maxillary Upper Premolar with an Immediate (Type 1) Implant.

General Factors	Assessment	Notes
Medical contraindications	None	
Smoking habit	None	
Growth considerations	None	
Site Factors	**Assessment**	**Notes**
Bone volume	Adequate, with intact socket walls	
Anatomic risk	Low	
Esthetic risk	Low	The patient had a low lip line
Complexity	Moderate	Careful preparation of the socket would be required Adjunctive bone augmentation could be required
Risk of complications	Moderate	Moderate risk of failing to gain ideal initial stability and proper axial alignment of the implant Slight risk of perforating the facial bone wall
SAC Classification	Advanced	

around the healing cap and secured in place with interrupted sutures (Figure 6). Healing progressed uneventfully, and restorative procedures commenced 8 weeks after surgery. At the 12 month postoperative review, the peri-implant tissues were healthy with stable crestal bone conditions (Figures 7 and 8).

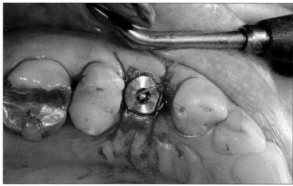

Figure 6.   Following connection of a healing cap, the flaps were closed with interrupted sutures to allow transmucosal healing.

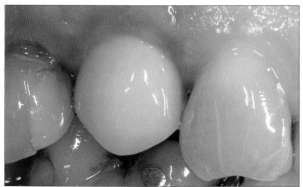

Figure 7.   Final implant-supported crown 12 months after surgery.

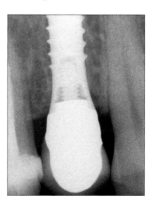

Figure 8.   Radiograph of the implant 12 months after surgery.

5 Classification of Restorative Cases

A. Dawson, W. Martin, U. Belser

5.1   Principles of Restorative Classification

The application of the SAC Classification to restorative cases will follow the general guidelines outlined below. These guidelines will assist in generating the normative classification of a clinical case type. Specific indications and the influence of modifying factors on these case types will be introduced in detail within this chapter.

Clinical cases may be assessed as *Straightforward, Advanced* or *Complex* when they meet the following criteria:

Straightforward
- A non-esthetic site, hence the esthetic risk is minimal.
- The restorative process is expected to be uncomplicated and involves few steps.
- The restorative outcome is readily predictable.
- There is a low risk of complications.

Advanced
- There is a discernable esthetic risk.
- The restorative process may have an increased number of steps, but the outcome is predictable.
- The restorative outcome can be accurately visualized.
- The risk of complications is low to moderate.

Complex
- The esthetic risk is moderate to high.
- The restorative process involves multiple steps, and the treatment plan may need to be re-evaluated as a consequence of the outcome of one or more of these steps.

- The restorative outcome cannot be readily visualized prior to treatment.
- The risk of complications is high, and multiple branching contingency plans may be necessary to deal with these issues. The long-term outcome of the restorative process may be compromised by these complications.
- Detailed coordination, communication, and sequencing of treatment procedures between the restorative dentist, surgeon and laboratory technician are essential for success. Patients must understand and accept the potential for compromised outcomes.

These criteria define the normative classification of case types. In addition, the Esthetic and Restorative modifying factors discussed in Chapter 3 may also apply in the risk assessment of specific cases. The following tables summarize the most significant of these modifying factors for each case type. These factors will be discussed below in the areas where they may have the greatest impact.

In general, factors such as the space available for restoration, the number of missing teeth to be replaced, and the quality and quantity of hard and soft tissues in the area will have an impact on the restorative classification.

5.2 Posterior Single Tooth Replacements

Table 1 summarizes the influence of specific modifying factors on the classification of posterior single tooth replacements. These modifying factors determine the normative classification for case types. These classifications can be adapted to fit specific situations by the restorative and esthetic factors discussed earlier. Users of the classification should look for the normative presentation that best fits their specific case and apply the necessary modifiers to obtain an appropriate SAC Classification.

Table 1. Modifying Factors for Posterior Single Tooth Replacement.

Posterior Single Tooth	Notes	Straightforward	Advanced	Complex
Inter-arch distance	Refers to the distance from the proposed implant restorative margin to the opposing occlusion	Ideal tooth height +/- 1 mm	Tooth height reduced by ≥ 2 mm	Non-restorable without adjunctive preparatory therapy due to severe over-eruption of opposing dentition
Mesio-distal space (Premolar)		Anatomic space corresponding to the missing tooth +/- 1 mm	Anatomic space corresponding to the missing tooth plus 2 mm or more.	Non-restorable without adjunctive preparatory therapy due to severe space restriction ≤ 5 mm
Mesio-distal space (Molar)		Anatomic space corresponding to the missing tooth +/- 1 mm	Anatomic space corresponding to the missing tooth +/- 2 mm or more	Non-restorable without adjunctive preparatory therapy due to severe space restriction ≤ 5 mm
Access		Adequate	Restricted	Access prohibits implant therapy
Loading protocol	To date, immediate restoration and loading procedures are lacking scientific documentation	Conventional or early	Immediate	
Esthetic risk	Refer to ERA (Treatment Guide 1)	Low	Moderate	Maxillary first premolars in patients with high esthetic demands
Occlusal para-function	Risk of complication to the restoration is high	Absent	Present	
Provisional implant-supported restorations	Situations where provisional restorations are recommended	Restorative margin < 3 mm apical to mucosal margin	Restorative margin > 3 mm apical to mucosal margin	

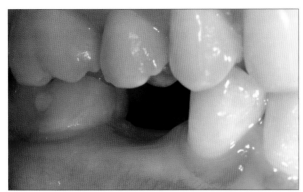

Figure 1.   Adequate inter-arch space for replacement of tooth 45.

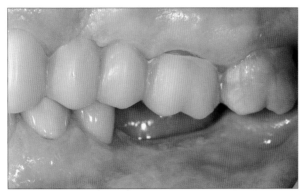

Figure 2.   Inadequate inter-arch space for replacement of tooth 36.

5.2.1   Space for Restoration

The inter-arch space available for restoration, which is the distance from the anticipated restorative margin to the opposing occlusal plane, will have an impact on the complexity of restorative treatment and the likelihood of complications (Figures 1 and 2). This issue may be less critical in bone-level implants where the shoulder of the implant is placed at the alveolar crest. These implant designs will often be accompanied by a wide selection of restorative components that allow for varying restorative margin positions. Implant designs that incorporate a transmucosal collar require planning that compensates for the height of the collar in situations where the inter-arch dimension is limited. In all implant designs, the space for restorative components and the ability to develop an ideal emergence profile are always critical. Restorative challenges are generally not associated with increased inter-arch space. Rather, limited inter-arch space is likely to complicate the process. When restorative space is limited, treatment plans will often include procedures to create ideal space. These procedures may include: adjustments to the opposing dentition, elective endodontics, crown lengthening, full-coverage restorations, orthodontic intrusion, or surgical osteotomies. Alternatively, when anatomy allows (e.g., when the inferior alveolar nerve position is favorable), the surgical plan may be modified to ensure that implants are placed more deeply to allow adequate space for restoration. However, such plans may result in deeply placed restorative margins that will indicate the use of screw-retained restorations.

Limited or excessive inter-arch space may influence esthetic outcomes, so special consideration must be given to patients who have any esthetic risk. Poor crown length-to-width ratios will have an adverse impact on esthetics. When crowns are too short, surgical management using deeper implant placement and soft tissue reduction techniques may be successful. However, esthetic compromises may still be evident in opposing arches where there is a mismatch in the sizes of restorations and natural teeth. Long crowns are often not easily managed without the assistance of vertical ridge augmentation or the use of tissue-colored porcelain.

The mesio-distal space available for restoration will also have an impact on the treatment regimen. Limited space, more often in premolar sites, may influence implant selection, surgical access, restorative materials and maintenance (Figures 3a to 3c). In patients with esthetic risk, restorative space limitations have an effect on crown proportions and interproximal soft tissue, often leading to an esthetic compromise. Situations with excessive mesio-distal space can also pose esthetic risk, and some form of adjunctive restorative treatment (such as modifying the contour of adjacent teeth with restorations or crowns) may be necessary.

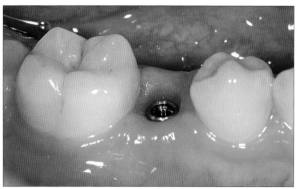

Figure 3a. Post-orthodontic result (tooth 45) with limited mesio-distal space (5 mm) requiring selection of a narrow platform implant.

5.2.2 Access

Restricted mouth opening may be a consequence of normal anatomy, temporomandibular joint problems, or other pathological conditions. This may limit the ability of surgeons and restorative dentists to gain access to a potential site for an implant-supported restoration. In general, this is most likely to be problematic in posterior sites, and may preclude implant treatment as an option. As a general rule, greater than 30 mm of inter-ach space is necessary for implant therapy.

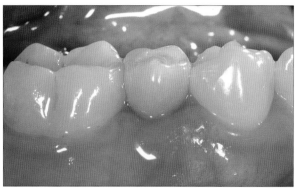

Figure 3b. Limited mesio-distal space (tooth 45), leading to compromised crown proportion and emergence profile when compared to adjacent teeth.

5.2.3 Loading Protocol

The Group 3 statements (Loading Protocols) from the Third ITI Consensus Conference (Cochran et al. 2004) recommended against employing immediate loading techniques in single tooth replacements, noting that at the time of the conference there was insufficient evidence to support this procedure as a routine technique in implant dentistry. Generally, this lack of supporting evidence is still an issue, although an increasing number of investigations are being conducted in this area of research. However, should immediate loading (i. e., occlusal loading of the implant via a provisional or definitive restoration within 48 hours of implant placement) be seen as desirable or necessary, it should be noted that this tends to place more stress on the treatment team. A higher level of expertise and logistic coordination are necessary compared to early or conventional loading protocols. Alternatively, immediate restoration (i. e., placement of a provisional restoration with no occlusal load within 48 hours of implant placement) may be utilized in situations where there is a high esthetic risk and/or a desire to maintain intra-arch space. In any event, care must be taken to prevent parafunctional non-axial loading of the dental implant.

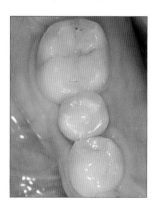

Figure 3c. Limited mesio-distal space (tooth 45), leading to compromised crown proportion and emergence profile when compared to adjacent teeth.

5.2.4   Esthetic Risk

In most cases, single tooth replacements in posterior sites will have little or no esthetic risk, and consequently are likely to have a normative restorative classification of *Straightforward*. However, in some situations where patients have high and broad smiles, premolar replacements (and occasionally those for molars) will have an assessable esthetic risk (Figure 4). In these cases, normative restorative classifications of *Advanced* or *Complex* may be appropriate.

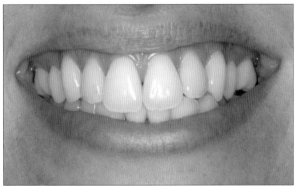

Figure 4.   Posterior tooth replacement would include an elevated esthetic risk in this patient with a high, broad smile.

5.2.5   Occlusal Parafunction

Current research suggests that, whereas implant failure is not increased by parafunctional overloading, the risk of technical complications such as screw loosening and fracture, abutment fracture, and loss of veneering materials is positively associated with parafunctional activity (Brägger et al. 2001). Thus, the presence of occlusal parafunction will increase the risk of complications and may make restorative procedures more demanding, and somewhat less predictable. The restorative dentist may need to modify the planned restoration to minimize potential effects of this overloading by using a retrievable restoration, or restorations employing veneering materials that are less prone to fracture, or softer materials that will result in less wear on the opposing dentition.

5.2.6   Provisional Restorations

When the placement of an implant-supported provisional restoration is indicated, the depth of the restorative platform beneath the mucosa will have an impact on the difficulty of this process. Implant shoulders located greater than 3 mm apical to the planned mucosal margin often require screw-retained or customized meso-structures that either eliminate the need for cementation, or move the cement margin to a position where access for removal of excess cement is readily available. Entrapment of cement within the peri-implant tissues can lead to undesirable inflammation, fistula formation, and in extreme situations, bone loss. Therefore, these case types should be considered *Advanced*.

5.3 Anterior Single Tooth Replacements

Table 1 demonstrates the most important factors in the assessment of single tooth replacements in anterior sites. As mentioned in Section 5.2, these variants will provide basic normative classifications that may need to be further amended based upon the influence of the modifying factors.

Table 1. Modifying Factors for Anterior Single Tooth Replacement.

Anterior Single Tooth	Notes	Straightforward	Advanced	Complex
Maxillomandibular relationship	Refers to horizontal and vertical overlap and the effect on restorability and esthetic outcome	Angle Class I and III	Angle Class II Div 1 and 2	Non-restorable without adjunctive preparatory therapy due to severe malocclusion
Mesio-distal space (maxillary central)	Symmetry is essential for successful outcome		Symmetry +/- 1 mm of contra-lateral tooth	Asymmetry greater than 1 mm
Mesio-distal space (maxillary laterals and canines)		Symmetry +/- 1 mm of contra-lateral tooth	Asymmetry greater than 1 mm	
Mesio-distal space (mandibular anterior)		Symmetry +/- 1 mm of contra-lateral tooth	Asymmetry greater than 1 mm	
Loading protocol	To date, immediate restoration and loading procedures are lacking scientific documentation	Conventional or early		Immediate
Esthetic risk	Refer to ERA (Treatment Guide 1)	Low	Moderate	High
Occlusal para-function	Risk of complication is to the restoration, not to implant survival	Absent		Present
Provisional implant-supported restorations	Provisional restorations are recommended		Restorative margin < 3 mm apical to mucosal margin	Restorative margin > 3 mm apical to mucosal margin

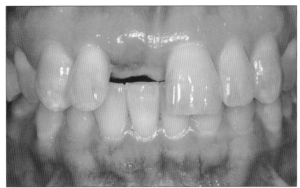

Figure 1a. Excessive vertical overlap, complicating replacement of tooth 11.

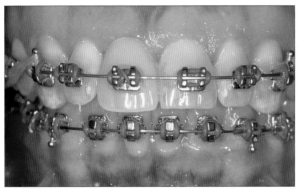

Figure 1b. Orthodontic therapy has been used to improve the vertical and horizontal relationship of the teeth.

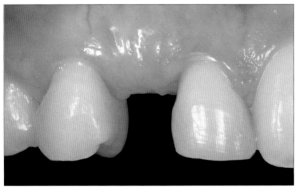

Figure 2a. Inadequate intra-arch space (6 mm) for replacement of tooth 13.

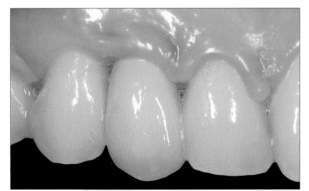

Figure 2b. A compromised peri-implant soft tissue result (tooth 13), even though adjacent tooth modification was performed in an attempt to increase intra-arch space.

5.3.1 Maxillomandibular Relationship

The anterior occlusal relationship, most importantly the degree of horizontal and vertical overlap, will influence the restorative difficulty and technical complications after treatment is complete. Space for restorative components can be restricted by these factors, as will be the loading vector on the final restoration. Deep bites with restricted horizontal overlap, such as those found in Angle Class II division 2 cases, are potentially the most problematic due to significant space restrictions as well as to the high potential for unfavorable loading vectors impacting the restorative materials, abutments and screws. The potential for adverse wear on opposing teeth must also be acknowledged. Often, adjunctive orthodontic treatment should be considered if implant-borne tooth replacements are desired (Figures 1a and 1b).

5.3.2 Mesio-Distal Space

Symmetry with the adjacent (central incisor) or contralateral (lateral incisor and canine) teeth can be one of the most important determinants of esthetic success in an implant restoration. This may well be a factor even in situations that are deemed to have low esthetic risk due to the smile line, because improper tooth proportions may still be visible. Maxillary central incisor replacements are most critical in this area, as the contralateral natural tooth is immediately adjacent to the implant restoration. Some increase in latitude for width discrepancy can be allowed for lateral incisor and canine replacements which are more distantly related to the comparison tooth. Similar latitude may be applied to lower anterior teeth, as they are less often visible. When the intra-arch space is inadequate, the limitation can have a negative impact on the implant selection, crown proportions and resulting interproximal soft tissues, potentially leading to an esthetic compromise (Figures 2a and 2b).

In situations with either a high esthetic need or demand, adjunctive orthodontic treatment or restorative intervention involving adjacent teeth may be necessary (Figure 3). This added complexity in the treatment would likely result in a classification of *Complex*.

5.3.3 Loading Protocol

As previously discussed, immediate loading protocols are currently not recommended for single tooth replacements. This is especially significant in the anterior region, where the risk of adverse esthetic outcomes is already an issue in many cases, even when conventional or early loading protocols are used. Additionally, the potential for significant non-axial loading of the implant may be a disadvantage during the healing period. Alternatively, immediate restoration of an implant may help improve the esthetic result by maintaining support of the peri-implant tissues and interproximal contact points at the time of surgery (Figures 4a to 4c). Implants possessing good primary stability in patients with favorable occlusal schemes that protect the provisional restoration during function could benefit from this technique. For these reasons, any immediate restorative procedure on single tooth implants in the anterior segment should be considered *Complex*.

5.3.4 Esthetic Risk

As discussed in Chapter 3, the level of esthetic risk can have a significant impact on the degree of difficulty of implant treatment in esthetic sites, as well as on the potential for adverse outcomes. Symmetry of the implant restoration with the surrounding teeth and tissues with respect to size, shape, color, and contour is crucial for achieving esthetic success. Consequently, issues that may reduce the likelihood of a successful outcome should be identified early in the assessment phase, and the patient advised of the impact that these issues may have on the outcome of treatment. While some anterior sites may be assessed as having low esthetic risk due to a low smile line or low esthetic demand, the majority of implant restorations in the anterior segments assume a moderate to high esthetic risk. Thus these cases will have classifications of at least *Advanced*. Currently, there is little evidence that allows us to accurately predict the soft-tissue outcome secondary to implant surgery, as well as the long-term stability of the peri-implant soft tissues. Thus, when the esthetic risk is high, and/or the patient's esthetic demands are high, the treatment regimen should be seen as *Complex*.

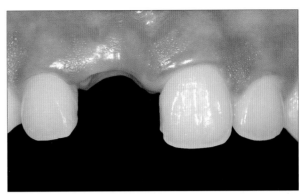

Figure 3. Increased mesio-distal dimension (tooth 11) when compared to the adjacent tooth, necessitating adjunctive treatment to achieve esthetic success.

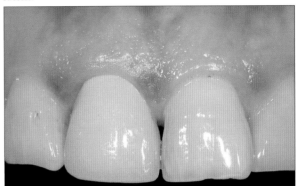

Figure 4a. Sub-osseous fracture of tooth 11 necessitating extraction of the tooth and placement of a dental implant.

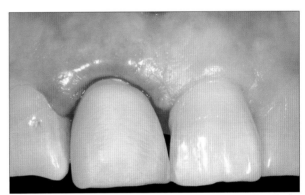

Figure 4b. Immediate implant placement with primary stability allowing for immediate restoration of tooth 11.

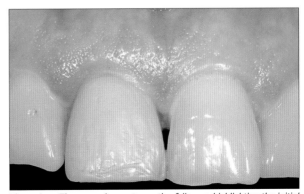

Figure 4c. The seven-day postoperative follow-up highlighting the initial maturation of the peri-implant tissues.

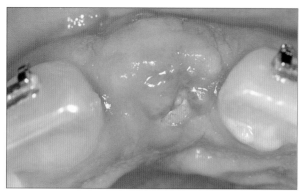

Figure 5a. Semi-submerged implant (tooth 21) requiring the fabrication of a provisional restoration.

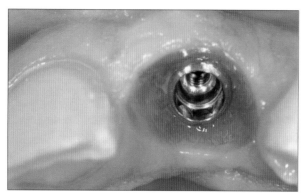

Figure 5b. Shaping of the transition zone accomplished with the provisional restoration over a four-week period.

5.3.5 Occlusal Parafunction

As noted previously, parafunctional loading of implant restorations can be associated with an increase in technical complications. In the anterior segment, while the amount of occlusal load is less than in posterior sites, the loading vector is more unfavorable due to a larger lateral component of this force. Overall, the potential for damage to the implant restoration and components such as abutments, screws, and restorative material remains significant in patients who practice a latero-protrusive form of bruxing, or those with excessive vertical overlap.

5.3.6 Provisional Restorations

Provisional implant-supported restorations are indicated in the anterior segment to develop the transition zone (the emergence created from the shoulder of the implant to the mucosal margin) and to prepare the site for the definitive restoration (Figures 5a and 5b). The three-dimensional position of the implant can influence the type of provisional restoration utilized (cemented vs. screw-retained). The depth of the implant shoulder below the mucosal margin and the patient's tissue biotype will affect the difficulty of the treatment and the predictability of the result. In the case of a deeply placed implant, the soft-tissue management is more demanding and the risk of complications is higher. In such situations, the need for screw retention and tissue shaping through multiple adjustments to the emergence profile of the provisional restoration cannot be overemphasized.

5.4 Posterior Extended Edentulous Spaces

Table 1 details the factors considered to influence the classification of multiple-tooth replacement restorations in posterior sites. Consideration of these factors, and any other modifiers such as those discussed in Chapter 3, will allow the classification of such cases.

Table 1. Modifying Factors for Posterior Extended Edentulous Space Restorations.

Posterior Extended Edentulous Spaces	Notes	Straightforward	Advanced	Complex
Esthetic risk	Refer for ERA (Treatment Guide 1)	Low	Moderate/High	
Access		Adequate	Restricted	Limited access does not allow for implant therapy
Inter-arch distance	Refers to the distance from the proposed implant restorative margin to the opposing occlusion	>8 mm	< 8 mm or >16 mm	
Mesio-distal space		Anatomic space corresponding to the missing teeth +/- 1 mm	Anatomic space corresponding to the missing teeth plus 2 mm or more, or space corresponding to a whole number of premolar units	Non-restorable without adjunctive preparatory therapy due to severe space restriction
Occlusion/ articulation		Harmonious	Irregular with no need for correction	Changes to existing occlusion necessary
Interim restorations during healing		None needed	Removable/ fixed	
Occlusal para-function	Risk of complication to the restoration is high.	Absent		Present
Loading protocol	To date, immediate restoration and loading procedures are lacking scientific documentation	Conventional or early	Immediate	
Cemented (Consensus Statement)		Accessible restorative margin	Sub-mucosal location of restorative margin	
Screw-retained		Multiple non-splinted Implants	Multiple splinted implants	

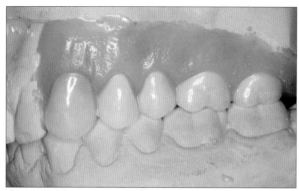

Figure 1a. Diagnostic wax-up of an extremely deficient quadrant as a result of a traumatic accident.

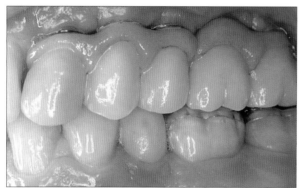

Figure 1b. Tissue-colored porcelain utilized to mask the remaining alveolar deficits following grafting and implant placement.

5.4.1   Esthetic Risk

The replacement of multiple teeth in posterior sites with implant restorations is not usually associated with significant esthetic risk, and such cases can normally be classified as *Straightforward*. However, in patients with excessively high or broad smiles (see Figure 4 in 5.2.4), these areas can be exposed, leading to a measurable esthetic risk and thus warranting classifications of *Advanced* or *Complex*. Edentulous ridges presenting with significant loss of hard and soft tissue contour may require either pre-surgical soft and hard tissue augmentation procedures or the use of tissue-colored porcelain to avoid excessively long teeth and to achieve acceptable esthetic outcomes (Figures 1a and 1b). These cases would likely be classified as having a moderate to high esthetic risk, and would have an overall classification of *Advanced*.

5.4.2   Access

Limited mouth opening can restrict access to posterior sites. This in turn may limit the number and type of implants which can be placed to support a multi-unit restoration. This often confines the location of these implants to more anterior positions where access is not as restricted. In some situations, restricted access will make implant placement impossible, and alternative tooth replacement techniques will be necessary.

5.4.3   Restorative Space

For restoration of an extended edentulous space in posterior segments, the ability to place ideal-sized restorations (i.e., those having dimensions similar to those of the teeth being replaced) will be associated with more straightforward techniques and can result in acceptable occlusal outcomes and esthetics. Drifting and tilting of adjacent teeth into these edentulous areas may restrict the restorative space to a dimension that is not consistent with that of the missing teeth, thus leading to less ideal outcomes if adjunctive therapies are not employed to create ideal space. In some situations, an acceptable compromise may be to restore these sites with reduced-size restorations that fill the space and create adequate contact points and embrasure forms to prevent food impaction. In these cases, modification or restoration of the adjacent teeth may be necessary. The most challenging situation involves a space that is either too wide or too narrow to allow these strategies to be used. Excessively wide restorations can compromise the peri-implant tissues, whereas narrow restorations can influence the material strength, often resulting in prosthesis fracture.

The vertical space available for restoration may be restricted due to a number of factors, such as loss of vertical dimension of occlusion, supra-eruption of opposing teeth, excessive wear, or small adjacent teeth. In these situations, placing the implant restorative shoulder deeper (when anatomic structures allow), or performing additional procedures to modify the opposing occlusal plane or increase occlusal vertical dimension, will be necessary to allow appropriate restoration of the dental implants (Figure 2). Excess vertical space is not normally problematic unless esthetic risk is also an issue. However, in some cases where excessively long crowns are necessary, it may be difficult to develop restoration contours that do not encourage food entrapment or make hygiene access more difficult for patients.

5.4.4 Occlusion and Parafunctional Habits

When posterior implant-supported restorations are protected by anterior guidance (mutually protected occlusion), or when they can be fabricated to prevent posterior guiding interferences, there will be a diminished risk of technical complications (retention screw loosening or fracture, abutment screw loosening or fracture, or fracture of the restoration veneering material). These situations would normally be *Straightforward*. However, when posterior restorations are involved in eccentric contacts, there is a greater non-axial load placed on implant components, and the risk of complications is increased. Such cases are classified as *Advanced* or *Complex*. The number of teeth to be replaced by such prostheses and the number of implants involved will be significant considerations in deriving classifications for such cases. For example, a four-unit fixed dental prosthesis (FDP) supported by two implants may be at higher risk of complications than a similarly situated three-unit FDP supported by two implants because of the different amounts of load placed on the prostheses.

As previously noted, occlusal parafunction increases the risk of technical complications. The presence of such habits may indicate specific treatment planning choices in the design of implant-supported FDPs for such cases. For example, more implants may be included in the design to provide better support, and the FDP might be screw retained rather than cement retained to allow removal of the prosthesis for repair. To reiterate, designing the occlusion on these prostheses to minimize eccentric contacts will be beneficial for the patient through reducing technical complications.

5.4.5 Interim Restorations During Healing

It is usually preferable to avoid using interim removable dental prostheses (RDPs) placed over healing implants, especially when they may apply uncontrolled loads on the implants during osseointegration. This contraindication is more relevant when dental implants are placed in a non-submerged position. When it is possible to avoid such RDPs, cases can be classified as *Straightforward*. If the interim restorations are necessary in order to fulfill patient desires or esthetic needs, preference should be given to tooth-supported restorations rather than those solely supported by the soft tissues. A simple, removable, tooth-supported interim restoration can be fabricated from 0.06-inch (1.5 mm) material vacuum-formed over a diagnostic cast, with acrylic resin teeth replacing the missing dental units. Alternatives might include a tooth-supported or temporary implant-supported FDP, or an RDP with a soft

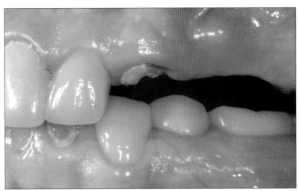

Figure 2. Limited inter-occlusal space to restore teeth 23 – 25 due to a loss of vertical dimension of occlusion.

lining. When an RDP is to be used, care should be taken to ensure that the saddle area over the implants is relieved to prevent any contact with the implant healing abutments. When an interim tooth replacement is planned, the additional steps involved in the process and the increased risk of complications indicate a classification of *Advanced*.

5.4.6 Loading Protocol

The Consensus Statements from the Third ITI Consensus Conference (Cochran et al. 2004) do not recommend the use of immediate loading protocols in partially edentulous cases. Conventional and early loading protocols are well documented and are not associated with additional risk. As such, a classification of *Straightforward* is appropriate. If immediate loading techniques are planned, however, the increased complexity and additional risk of complications necessitate a classification of at least *Advanced*.

5.4.7 Prosthesis Retention System

The decision on whether to retain an implant restoration with cement or screws is based on a number of factors, including the operator's preference, cost, implant position, and the need for retrievability. Each option, however, has specific considerations which will have an impact on the degree of difficulty of the process and the risk of complications.

Cemented implant restorations can provide an easy and effective means of retention that avoids some of the pitfalls associated with screw retention. Cemented restorations normally fit passively, and there is no potential for screw access holes to compromise esthetics, weaken porcelain, or interfere with occlusion. However, inaccessi-

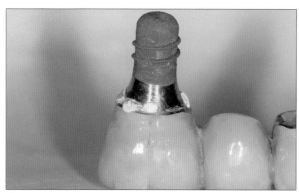

Figure 3.   Implant failure as a consequence of peri-implantitis associated with sub-mucosal cement deposits.

ble cement from a deeply placed implant restorative margin may be associated with an increased risk of peri-implant complications (Figure 3). Thus, when the restoration margin for a cemented restoration is placed sub-mucosally and access for removal of excess cement is limited, a classification of *Advanced* should be applied.

Screw retention results in closer marginal adaptation (Keith et al. 1999), which is preferable when the restorative margin is placed sub-mucosally. In situations where multiple implants will be splinted, the need for framework passivity is magnified when screw retention is desired. Here, significant strain may result (Karl et al. 2008), leading to technical complications such as fracture of restoration veneering materials. Clinical impression and verification techniques are often employed to help achieve this accurate fit of the framework. Due to this increased difficulty, cases should be classified as *Advanced* if multiple splinted screw-retained restorations are planned.

5.5 Anterior Extended Edentulous Spaces

Table 1 summarizes the factors considered to influence the classification of multiple-tooth replacement in anterior sites. Consideration of these factors, and any other modifiers such as those discussed in Chapter 3, will allow the classification of such cases.

Table 1. Modifying Factors for Anterior Extended Edentulous Space Restorations.

Anterior Extended Edentulous Spaces	Notes	Straightforward	Advanced	Complex
Esthetic risk	Refer for ERA (Treatment Guide 1)	Low	Moderate	High
Intermaxillary relationship	Refers to horizontal and vertical overlap and the effect on restorability and esthetic outcome	Class I and III	Class II Div 1 and 2	Non-restorable without adjunctive preparatory therapy due to severe malocclusion
Mesio-distal space		Adequate for required tooth replacement	Insufficient space available for replacement of all missing teeth	Adjunctive therapy necessary to replace all missing teeth
Occlusion/ articulation		Harmonious	Irregular, with no need for correction	Changes of existing occlusion necessary
Interim restorations during healing		RDP	Fixed	
Provisional implant-supported restorations	Provisional restorations are recommended		Restorative margin <3 mm apical to mucosal crest	Restorative margin >3 mm apical to mucosal crest
Occlusal parafunction	Risk of complication is to the restoration, not to implant survival	Absent		Present
Loading protocol	To date, immediate restoration and loading procedures are lacking scientific documentation	Conventional or early		Immediate

5.5.1 Esthetic Risk

The degree of esthetic risk in cases involving multiple-tooth replacements in anterior sites will likely be the major determinant of the SAC Classification. Factors hindering the restorative dentist from developing symmetry with contralateral tooth segments and from achieving pleasing soft-tissue contours will increase the degree of difficulty in these cases. This will be mirrored in the classification level. Some of these factors are discussed below. A detailed discussion of all criteria can be found in Volume 1 of the ITI Treatment Guide (Martin et al. 2007).

Soft tissue contour. Achieving pleasing soft-tissue outcomes can be highly problematic where multiple adjacent teeth have been lost and the hard- and soft-tissue contours have been altered by the resorptive process. Of special consideration is the ability to develop the appearance of symmetrical papillae in these sites. When teeth are present, the inter-dental papilla is supported by the periodontal attachment (supra-crestal fibers) of the teeth, and will indicate the "ideal" that is to be achieved. However, as no such support is available adjacent to multiple implants, alternative methods of developing esthetic soft tissue contours are necessary. Soft- and/or hard-tissue

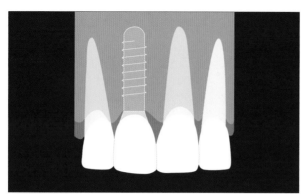

Figure 1a.   Diagram of a single tooth implant. The periodontal attachment on the adjacent teeth provides support to the papillae between the implant and adjacent teeth.

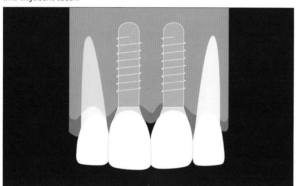

Figure 1b.   Diagram of two adjacent implants showing blunting of the papilla between the two implants due to loss of crestal bone height, and formation of a dark triangle apical to the contact area.

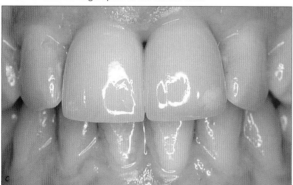

Figure 1c and 1d.   Adjacent implant restorations in the 11 and 21 sites. Note the blunting of the midline papilla. The radiograph demonstrates the reduced inter-implant bone height.

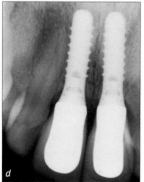

augmentation, tissue shaping techniques such as ovate pontics, or soft tissue replacements like tissue-colored porcelain will be necessary to imitate papillae between these restorations. Where artificial soft-tissues are used, the need to mask the junction between these and the natural tissues will result in additional complexity. In general, extended edentulous spaces will often require augmentation procedures to enhance the contours of the resorbed ridges in order to achieve esthetically acceptable outcomes. The complexity of these processes, and the difficulty in predicting the treatment outcome, will generally lead to classifications of *Advanced* or *Complex* in cases where there is any discernable esthetic risk.

Adjacent implants. It has been demonstrated (Tarnow et al. 2000) that insufficient space between adjacent implants results in decreased papillary height, and subsequently in compromised esthetic outcomes (Figures 1a to 1d). These outcomes can be magnified in situations in which restricted mesio-distal space prevents adequate spacing of implant platforms. A minimum of 3 mm between implant platforms is considered necessary to maintain papilla height when implants are placed adjacent to each other. A commonly used alternative is the cantilevered implant restoration. These are often indicated when a lateral incisor replacement is involved (i.e., canine-lateral or central-lateral) utilizing an ovate pontic (Figures 2a and 2b). Notwithstanding this, cases where adjacent implants may be necessary will normally attract a classification of *Complex* when the esthetic needs of the case are moderate to high.

5.5.2   Intermaxillary Relationships

As noted in section 5.3.1, the horizontal and vertical occlusal relationships in anterior sites may restrict the space for restorative components and subject restorations and retentive elements to significant non-axial loads. Angle Class I anterior occlusions with minimal horizontal and vertical overlap, and Angle Class III occlusions with an edge-to-edge incisal relationship, pose the lowest risk of these difficulties, and hence earn a classification of *Straightforward*. Deeper bites, and those with restricted horizontal space such as Angle Class II division 2 malocclusions, are at much greater risk of treatment difficulty and of technical complications, and thus should be classified as at least *Advanced*.

5.5.3   Restorative Space Issues

In the anterior segment, there will generally be a need to achieve symmetry of tooth width irrespective of the lip line at smile, as the incisal edges of anterior teeth are usually visible during speech and at rest. Thus, the mesio-distal width necessary for a symmetrical restoration to the adjacent or contra-lateral teeth will generally be dictated by this need. When a minor asymmetry is present compared with contralateral teeth, restorations may need to be designed that incorporate minor modifications to give the appearance of symmetry. These situations will normally be identified during the completion of trial set-ups and interim restorations for these cases. The final tooth positions can then be reproduced in the final restoration. In severe cases of space mismatch, adjunctive treatments such as orthodontics or adjusting the contours of adjacent teeth through odontoplasty, or placing bonded restorations or crowns, may be necessary (Figure 3). *Straightforward* cases will be those in which little additional planning or treatment is needed to achieve an acceptable result. An increased need for additional intervention, or an increased risk of a compromised esthetic result, will lead to classifications of *Advanced* or *Complex*.

5.5.4 Occlusion/Articulation

Harmonious tooth arrangements in these segments will generally carry a lower risk of esthetic compromise and will normally be classed as *Straightforward*. When there is a need for tooth replacements to fit into complex occlusal schemes where crowding, wear, cross-bites, tilting of teeth, or irregular occlusal planes exist, the risk of compromised esthetic outcomes is increased. As such, the SAC Classification level will also increase in complexity. More complex occlusal situations are also more likely to provide insufficient space for components. Additionally, these arrangements may result in non-axial loading of implants. These factors will generally be associated with greater risk of technical complications. In cases where the occlusion is severely compromised, additional treatment steps, such as orthodontics or more extensive restorative rehabilitation, may be necessary. In these cases, a classification of *Complex* is appropriate.

5.5.5 Interim Restorations During Healing

In most esthetic cases, some form of interim tooth replacement will be necessary during the healing period. These restorations can be used to trial the esthetic outcomes planned for the case, assist in shaping of the tissues during healing, and serve as a template for the final restorations. However, the risk of such provisional restorations placing uncontrolled loads on integrating implants cannot be discounted, and care must be taken to minimize this risk.

RDPs provide the simplest provisional restorations for these cases, assuming care is taken to ensure that the pontic does not load the implants underneath it during healing. Vacuum-formed retainers offer the ability to keep

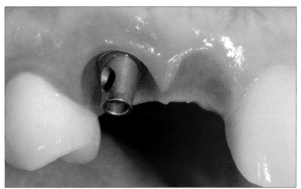

Figure 2a. A dental implant in site 13 to support a restoration replacing 12 and 13.

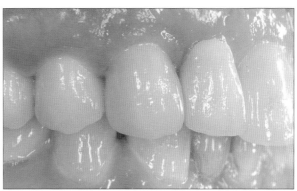

Figure 2b. A restoration on implant 13 utilizing a mesial cantilever in site 12.

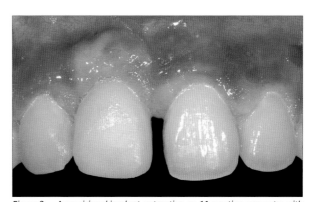

Figure 3. A provisional implant restoration on 11 creating symmetry with 21. The patient desires to close the diastema. A restoration on the mesial aspect of 21 will be needed, in addition to a wider definitive restoration on 11, to maintain symmetry.

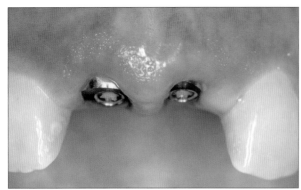

Figure 4a.   Dental implants in sites 11 and 21 prior to loading.

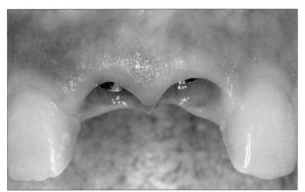

Figure 4b.   Shaped transition zone established after four weeks using implant-supported provisional restorations.

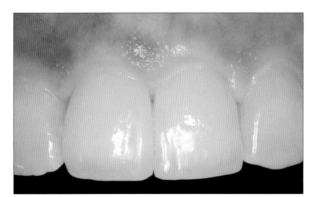

Figure 4c.   Definitive implant restorations on 11 and 21, resulting in an acceptable esthetic result.

pressure off the tissues while utilizing the surrounding teeth for support. FDPs can also be used to provide provisional tooth replacements during this period. These may be supported by teeth or by provisional implants. The increased complexity of the processes associated with fixed provisional restorations leads to a classification of at least *Advanced*.

5.5.6   Provisional Implant-Supported Restorations

Provisional restorations placed on implants at the time of implant placement or following integration are critical in establishing support for the peri-implant tissues to form an adequate transition zone for the definitive restorations. This approach will assist in developing esthetically pleasing soft tissue architecture surrounding implants or in pontic sites, and can lead to better esthetic outcomes (Figures 4a to 4c). This process requires skill and patience, and is normally classified as *Advanced*. When the restorative margin for the implant is more than 3 mm below the mucosal margin, this process becomes technically more difficult, and should be classified as *Complex*.

5.5.7   Occlusal Parafunction

Given the risks of technical complications in patients with parafunctional habits, and as non-axial loading is the norm in the anterior segment, a classification of *Complex* will be associated with any case in which there is a significant parafunctional habit. These risks are especially important in patients who practice a latero-protrusive form of bruxism. Utilization of an occlusal nightguard is recommended in patients with these tendencies.

5.5.8   Loading Protocol

Little comment on this topic is necessary beyond that made in earlier parts of this chapter. However, it is worth noting that the loading vectors in the anterior segment, and especially in the anterior maxilla, tend to diminish the chances of success in immediate loading for extended anterior restorations. These cases often lack sufficient occlusal contacts on adjacent teeth to provide any protection for these implants. This increases the likelihood that excessive loading will result in failure of the implants to osseointegrate. A classification of *Complex* is thus associated with any immediate loading treatment. When sufficient occlusal protection exists in the surrounding dentition, immediate restoration of the dental implants can be performed, and may help to expedite the shaping of the transition zone. This therapy would carry a classification ranging from *Advanced* to *Complex*, depending on the position and number of dental implants involved.

5.6 Edentulous Maxilla – Fixed Prosthesis

Table 1 summarizes the factors that have the most influence on the classification of full-arch fixed restorations in the maxilla. The classification of a specific case is based on these factors in combination with the other restorative modifiers discussed in Chapter 3. In general, the normative classification of fixed maxillary full-arch restorations is at least *Advanced*.

Table 1. Modifying Factors for the Edentulous Maxillary Presentation – Fixed Prosthesis.

Edentulous Maxilla – Fixed	Notes	Straightforward	Advanced	Complex
Inter-arch distance	Refers to the distance from the proposed implant restorative margin to the opposing occlusion. Note: hybrid restorations will need more space.		Average	Space restricted for adequate restoration
Access			Adequate	Restricted
Loading protocol	To date, immediate restoration and loading procedures are lacking scientific documentation		Conventional or early	Immediate
Esthetic risk	Refer for ERA (Treatment Guide 1)		Low	Moderate/high
Interim restorations during healing			Removable	Fixed
Occlusal para-function	Risk of complication is to the restoration, not to implant survival		Absent	Present
Occlusal scheme/ issues			Anterior guidance	No anterior guidance

5.6.1   Restorative Space Issues

Inter-arch space will likely be the most important technical consideration in these restorative cases. The space required for abutments, frameworks and restorative materials has a great impact in this area. The available space for restoration is determined prior to the commencement of treatment through the use of the remaining dentition or interim restorations, and in the case of the edentulous arch, through a wax setup of the denture teeth. It is imperative to understand that different fixed-restorative techniques will have different space requirements. Restorative procedures that employ denture teeth and acrylic resin tissue supported by metal (gold alloy or titanium) frameworks (often referred to as Hybrid restorations) will require more vertical space (for the components, framework and denture teeth with veneering material) than those using porcelain-fused-to-metal (PFM) restorations. The former techniques will require at least 10 mm to 15 mm of space between the restorative platform and the opposing occlusion, while the PFM restorations can be utilized in more restricted spaces with a minimum inter-ach distance of 7 mm to 8 mm.

Unfavorable resorptive patterns of the hard and soft tissues in the maxilla can lead to limitations in the oro-facial placement of the dental implants. In the absence of augmentation procedures, the potential for palatal placement of dental implants increases with the degree of maxillary atrophy. Situations with limited interocclusal space and palatal placement of the dental implants could lead to such restorative complications as prosthesis and/or framework fracture, poor emergence profile, ridge-lap restorations, inadequate lip support, limitations to access for home maintenance procedures, and interference with phonetics. Attention to detail is critical when evaluating edentulous patients for maxillary fixed restorations, as improper planning and placement of the dental implants will result in compromises that will require continual maintenance. Due to these factors, it is recommended that treatment of the edentulous maxilla with restricted space for restoration carry a classification of *Complex*.

5.6.2   Access

Restricted mouth opening may complicate or even completely preclude implant placement or restoration. This will be most critical in posterior sites. During initial assessment, measurement of the available space to ensure adequate access for surgical and restorative instrumentation, as well as prosthetic components and final restorations, may be indicated. In general, this distance will become easier to achieve as arches become edentulous.

5.6.3   Loading Protocol

While there is a higher potential for non-axial loading on implants placed in the edentulous maxilla, the immediate loading of implants with a splinted, passive fitting restoration can have favorable results (Ibañez et al. 2005). In such situations, a greater complexity is associated with this procedure due to a higher risk of complications in the planning, fabrication and delivery of the prosthesis. Therefore, immediate loading of fixed maxillary full-arch restorations is generally considered *Complex*.

5.6.4   Esthetic Risk

In the planning of a full-arch prosthesis, the fabrication of an interim denture with ideal tooth positioning and lip support is mandatory when the existing denture is deemed inadequate for proper esthetic diagnosis and planning. This interim denture will assist in fabrication of a radiographic and surgical template that will indicate planned implant positions in relation to the final tooth positions. It will also serve as a tool to determine the patient's suitability for a definitive fixed restoration. The lip support provided by the flange of the denture will need to be addressed if a fixed restoration is desired. In some situations, this may be the factor determining whether a hybrid restoration or an implant overdenture is the definitive restoration. If a fixed result is desired in areas of inadequate lip support, significant grafting will be needed to rebuild the horizontal deficiency and allow for proper implant positioning and emergence profile of the restoration.

The need for soft tissue replacement in maxillary full-arch cases can have a significant impact on the esthetic risk of the treatment. The ability of the practitioner and technician to hide the junction between the prosthetic soft tissues and the mucosal ridge will dictate the level of difficulty of such cases. The height of the lip line and smile will influence this ability (Figures 1a and 1b).

When sufficient ridge volume remains to avoid the need for soft and hard tissue replacement, the coincidence of implant position with "roots" of replacement teeth will be the most critical esthetic issue. In other words, maintaining embrasure form is essential to esthetic success, and placement of the dental implants within the confines of tooth position is extremely important to establish proper contours and symmetry of the restorations. Acceptable esthetic results will normally be achieved if this goal is realized. However, if this goal cannot be achieved, or if final implant placements fall short of this ideal in the esthetic zone, compromised esthetic outcomes will ensue. Positioning of the dental implants within these embrasures is less critical in situations in which soft-tissue replacements are necessary, as these pink porcelain or resin flanges will mask deficiencies. Treatment of the edentulous maxilla with fixed restorations in patients with medium to high esthetic risk is often associated with procedures that carry added complexity and therefore increase the classification from *Advanced* to *Complex*.

5.6.5 Interim Restorations During Healing

In situations when immediate loading of the dental implants has not been pursued, a conventional maxillary interim denture will likely be used during implant healing. There is moderate risk of uncontrolled loads being placed on healing implants via this prosthesis, so care must be taken to minimize this risk. Placement of the implants in a submerged fashion, coupled with a soft liner relieved in the areas over the implants, will help minimize complications.

In some instances, an interim FDP may be utilized when remaining teeth (to be replaced by the final full-arch prosthesis) are sufficiently robust. This FDP can be placed in the arch to support the restoration while the implants osseointegrate. Temporary implants can also be indicated in situations that lack adequate natural tooth support for the interim restoration. Fixed interim restorations carry some benefits over the removable prosthesis, and should be explored when possible. However, the increased complexity and risk of these treatments would normally entail a classification of *Complex*.

5.6.6 Occlusal Parafunction

Occlusal parafunction has the potential to damage the implant-supported prostheses through excessive wear or fracture. When such habits exist, the risk of complications is much higher, as is the need for maintenance. Such cases would normally have a classification of *Complex*.

The occlusal scheme of the final prosthesis will have an influence on final outcomes and stability of the restoration and temporomandibular joints. When establishing the final occlusal scheme, elimination of non-working interferences is essential to long-term stability of the fixed restoration. A balanced occlusal scheme is only pursued if the opposing arch possesses a removable prosthesis. A group function occlusal scheme may have somewhat greater potential for wear and restoration fracture than a mutually protected approach. Thus, these types of occlusal scheme may be classified as being more complex than the norm.

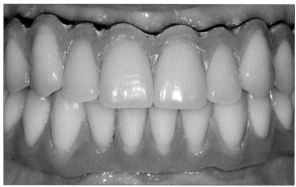

Figure 1a. A maxillary Hybrid restoration highlighting the joint between the prosthesis and tissue.

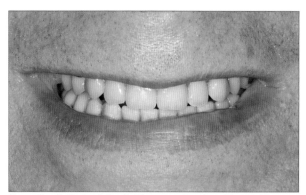

Figure 1b. Patient at full smile. The mucosal borders of the Hybrid restoration are hidden.

5.7   Edentulous Mandible – Fixed Prosthesis

Table 1 outlines the significant modifying factors most applicable to the fixed, full-arch restoration in the mandible. While the normative classification for this case type is *Advanced*, a number of factors may increase the difficulty of treatment to a level where a classification of *Complex* is more appropriate.

Table 1. Modifying Factors for the Edentulous Mandible – Fixed Prosthesis.

Edentulous Mandible – Fixed	Notes	Straightforward	Advanced	Complex
Inter-arch distance	Refers to the distance from the proposed implant restorative margin to the opposing occlusion. Note: hybrid restorations will need more space.		Adequate	Excessive (mechanical leverage issues) or restricted (space for components)
Loading protocol	To date, immediate restoration and loading procedures are lacking scientific documentation		Conventional/early	Immediate
Esthetic risk	Refer for ERA (Treatment Guide 1)		Low	Moderate/high
Interim restorations during healing			Removable	Fixed
Occlusal para-function	Risk of complication is to the restoration, not to implant survival		Absent	Present
Occlusal scheme/ issues			Anterior guidance	No anterior guidance

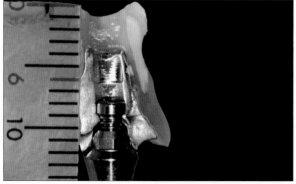

Figure 1.   A cross section of a mandibular Hybrid, highlighting the inter-arch space needed for components, framework, denture teeth and acrylic resin.

5.7.1   Restorative Space Issues

In most circumstances, there will be adequate space available for restorative implant components and restorations. As in the maxillary arch, the mandibular Hybrid prosthesis will require a greater amount of space, especially with respect to inter-arch distance and bulk in the oro-facial dimension, than prostheses fabricated using metal ceramic techniques (Figure 1). Hybrid prostheses do, however, have some advantages with respect to laboratory procedures and a lower risk of framework distortion during fabrication. Additionally, repairs to Hybrid prostheses are generally more easily undertaken and can often be performed at the chairside.

Excessive inter-arch distance can be associated with increased risk of technical complications as a consequence of the mechanical disadvantage imposed by this type of arrangement, in which the occlusal contact is distant from the restoration's base of support. Another factor that contributes to this risk is the non-axial loading that is often associated with long cantilever extensions distal to the posterior implants when implant sites are not available distal to the mental foramen. Generally, the implants in these situations are placed at the crest of the residual ridge, where the bone height is favorable and the surrounding mucosa is keratinized. Given that the pattern of bone resorption in edentulous ridges tends to result in a lingual migration of the ridge, the teeth on these FDPs often must be placed more facially to achieve ideal esthetic and functional outcomes. This can result in significant non-axial load vectors, which may unfavorably impact screws and screw joints. Such cases are best classified as *Complex* for these reasons.

5.7.2 Loading Protocol

The statements from the Third ITI Consensus Conference (Cochran et al. 2004) note that there is a reasonable amount of evidence supporting the immediate loading of fixed mandibular prostheses supported by a minimum of four implants. This protocol provides some advantages, as it eases the transition for the patient from having some remaining teeth to a complete implant-supported "dentition" in the mandible, and also avoids the potential for uncontrolled loading of integrating implants via interim complete dentures. However, the added complexity of this process with respect to the logistics of organizing this type of treatment in the traditional "implant team" treatment approach, and the increased difficulty of the clinical procedures, indicate that a classification of *Complex* is most appropriate.

5.7.3 Esthetic Risk

In most cases there is little esthetic risk involved in the mandible, and the normative classification of *Advanced* is usually appropriate. However, when there is any measurable esthetic risk, the additional complexity of the resulting treatment will justify a classification of *Complex*.

5.7.4 Interim Restorations During Healing

As previously noted, there is a potential for complete dentures to place uncontrolled loads on implants during the healing phase. This is perhaps most problematic in the mandible, where denture instability and poor retention are virtually the norm. In such cases the risk of complications indicates a classification of *Advanced*. These latter problems can be avoided using immediate loading techniques, or by using some retained teeth or temporary implants to support fixed provisional restorations. These ad-

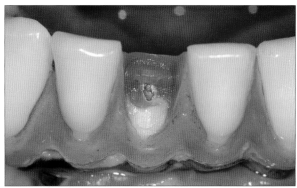

Figure 2. Fracture of a denture tooth on a Hybrid restoration in a patient with occlusal parafunctional habits.

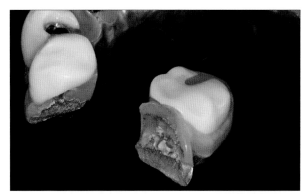

Figure 3. Fracture of a Hybrid restoration's distal extension. The fracture was a result of inadequate framework thickness in a patient with limited inter-arch space for restoration and occlusal parafunctional habits.

ditional procedures increase the complexity and risk, and warrant a classification of *Complex*.

5.7.5 Occlusal Parafunction

When present, occlusal parafunctional habits will increase the risk of technical complications with fixed prostheses, thus indicating a classification of *Complex*. Wear may also be a significant issue, especially when resin-based veneering materials have been utilized. However, resin-based materials may be the material of choice in such cases, as they are more easily modified and repaired than metal and ceramic materials (Figure 2).

The occlusal scheme will also have an impact on wear and on the potential for technical complications (Figure 3). Schemes that employ some anterior guidance with elimination of occlusal interferences will have somewhat less potential for damage. Where group-function schemes are employed, the potential for wear and veneering material fracture is increased. Balanced or lingualized occlusal schemes are of merit in situations where the opposing arch is restored with a conventional complete denture.

5.8 Edentulous Maxilla – Removable Prosthesis

The normative classification for maxillary implant-supported/retained overdentures is *Advanced*. Table 1 summarizes the most significant restorative modifying factors. It should be noted that overdentures tend to be associated with higher rates of technical and biological complications and require more maintenance than other restoration types (Berglundh et al. 2002), thus supporting the *Advanced* normative classification.

Table 1. Modifying Factors for the Edentulous Maxilla – Removable Prosthesis.

Edentulous Maxilla – Removable	Notes	Straightforward	Advanced	Complex
Inter-arch distance (bar & clip retained)	Refers to the distance from the proposed implant restorative margin to the opposing occlusion.		> 10 mm	< 10 mm = not indicated
Inter-arch distance (Individual retentive elements)			> 8 mm	< 8 mm = not indicated
Loading protocol (bar & clip retained)			Early	Immediate (bar only)
Loading protocol (individual retentive elements)			Conventional/Early	
Esthetic risk	Refer for ERA (Treatment Guide 1)		Low	Moderate/high (unrealistic expectations)
Interim restorations during healing			Removable	
Occlusal para-function	Risk of complication is to the restoration, not to implant survival		Absent	Present
Occlusal scheme/issues (fixed opposing arch)			Anterior guidance	No anterior guidance
Occlusal Scheme/Issues (Complete denture in opposing arch)			Balanced	Balanced occlusion not possible

5.8.1   Restorative Space

Implant overdentures are the most space-demanding restoration designs, especially when bar and clip retentive features are utilized. The bulk of implant components and retentive elements that have to be confined within the denture housing is significant, and can often be a contributing factor in weakening of the denture. In such cases, cast-metal reinforcing frameworks are often indicated (Figure 1). In situations without sufficient inter-arch space, alternative restoration designs or surgical procedures to create space may need to be considered.

In most situations, maxillary overdentures will involve four or more implants for retention and support. These situations dictate that such prostheses are predominantly implant supported, indicating that splinting of implants using bar assemblies may be selected, especially when implant axis or positioning is compromised. These bar and clip designs occupy the most volume in the final prostheses, and usually require cast-metal reinforcement of the denture to retain adequate strength. When near-parallel implants of satisfactory length are possible, Locator™ (Zest Anchors, Escondido, CA, USA) or o-ring retention systems can be used. These attachments occupy less inter-arch space and overall volume, and therefore can be used in cases where restorative space is restricted (Figure 2). Non-splinted implants can also be used with magnetic retention systems, and may be useful where parallelism is not possible. However, these retention systems tend to require more inter-arch space and volume than other non-splinted systems (but possibly less space than bar-clip designs), and generally do not achieve the same retention as the mechanical retention systems.

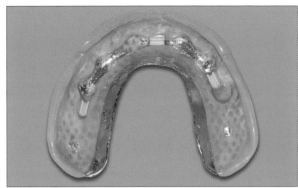

Figure 1.   An open palate maxillary overdenture with a cast-metal reinforcing framework.

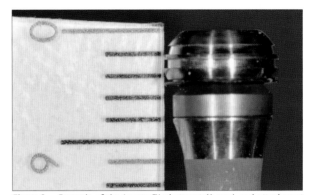

Figure 2.   Example of the Locator™ abutment (1 mm) and attachment height.

5.8.2   Loading Protocol

Immediate loading of implants in the maxilla with an overdenture is not recommended as a routine procedure by the Third ITI Consensus Conference (Cochran et al. 2004). Where this protocol is to be used, rigid splinting of the implants with a bar assembly is necessary. The increased complexity and risk of such procedures indicates a classification of *Complex*. Immediate loading of non-splinted implants in the maxilla is currently not recommended in any situation.

5.8.3   Esthetic Risk

In general, an implant-retained/supported overdenture will not improve the esthetic outcome any more than a conventional complete denture. A natural appearance of the acrylic-resin base can be enhanced through customized tissue characterization, but it should be noted in situations with limited material thickness that masking of the underlying components can become difficult. Thus patients must be made aware of these limitations prior to treatment. If patients have esthetic needs or desires that cannot realistically be met by these techniques, alternative procedures may be indicated. If overdentures are to be used in these high-esthetic-risk cases, a classification of *Complex* is appropriate.

5.8.4   Interim Restorations During Healing

Interim maxillary dentures will likely be necessary throughout the healing period and during the design and fabrication of the definitive prosthesis. Care must be taken to avoid any uncontrolled loading of the implants during the healing phase through the use of soft-liners and selective relief over the implant healing abutments. When possible, placing healing abutments that are flush with the mucosa will minimize the unfavorable forces that could cause failure of the implants to osseointegrate.

5.8.5   Occlusal Parafunction

Parafunctional habits will increase the risk of technical complications and the need for maintenance visits. In general, implant-retained/supported overdentures are continually subjected to movement between the retentive components and the bar or abutments, as supporting soft tissues compress under load. This movement results in attachment wear, and can be associated with component fracture. Consequently, the need for maintenance (by way of replacing worn or broken retentive elements) is increased when compared with fixed implant-supported restorations. Occlusal parafunction, which will increase load as well as the frequency of these loading cycles, will hasten this wear and increase the risk of fracture, resulting in greater maintenance needs.

Planning of the occlusal scheme for the overdenture should focus on the restorative status of the opposing dentition. In situations where the opposing arch is restored with an overdenture or conventional denture, a balanced or lingualized occlusal scheme should be incorporated. Where the opposing arch is natural dentition or restored teeth/implants, the occlusal scheme should center on the weakest arch (in this situation the maxillary overdenture), also indicating a balanced or lingualized occlusal scheme. Attention should be paid to the potential for increased wear rates of the denture teeth and attachments.

5.9 Edentulous Mandible – Removable Prosthesis

The normative classification for implant overdentures in the mandible can be as low as *Straightforward* for the two-implant overdenture. However, greater numbers of implants, and a movement towards significant implant support of the prosthesis, will tend to shift the classification of these cases to *Advanced*. As in the maxillary overden-ture, implant-supported/retained overdentures in the mandible tend to be associated with higher rates of biological and technical complications, and require greater amounts of maintenance than do fixed implant restorations. Table 1 outlines the influence of the more important modifying factors for this treatment type.

Table 1. Modifying Factors for the Edentulous Mandible – Removable Prosthesis.

Edentulous Mandible – Removable	Notes	Straightforward	Advanced	Complex
Inter-arch distance (bar & clip retained)	Refers to the distance from proposed implant restorative margin to opposing occlusion.		> 10 mm	< 10 mm = not indicated
Inter-arch distance (individual retentive elements)		> 8 mm		< 8 mm = not indicated
Number of implants		2	3 or more	
Loading protocol		Conventional/ early		Immediate
Esthetic risk	Refer for ERA (Treatment Guide 1)	Low	Moderate/high (unre-alistic expectations)	
Interim restorations during healing		Removable		
Occlusal para-function	Risk of complication is to the restoration, not implant survival		Absent	Present
Occlusal scheme/issues (fixed opposing arch)			Anterior guidance	No anterior guidance
Occlusal scheme/issues (complete denture in opposing arch)			Balanced	Balanced occlusion not possible

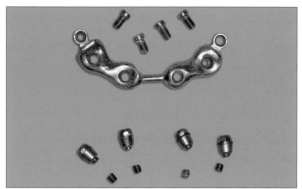

Figure 1.   Fractured abutment screws used in a patient with severe para-functional habits.

5.9.1   Restorative Space

The edentulous mandible resorbs at a greater rate than the maxilla, and will therefore often allow for adequate restorative space for abutments, bars and retentive elements. Patients who are undergoing extractions in preparation for overdentures may benefit from alveoloplasty procedures to create sufficient space for these components and prevent restorative complications. In situations with limited restorative space, consideration should be given to incorporating denture frameworks as well as utilizing individual attachments (i.e., Locator™). As mentioned earlier, bar and clip designs require the greatest amount of space with regard to both the inter-arch distance and the overall volume of components that must be included within the confines of the denture. Fortunately, the recent success of the Locator™ attachment (which requires the least space) has led to this being the attachment of choice in the mandibular overdenture. Any significant impingement of these prostheses into the patient's tongue space (as a result of this bulk, or as a consequence of sub-optimal implant placement) can result in comfort, functional and phonetic difficulties.

5.9.2   Number of Implants

Mandibular overdentures supported by two implants gain retention and stability from the implant attachments while being predominantly tissue supported. They are placed in simple procedures that carry a relatively low risk of complications. Consequently, these cases are normally classified as *Straightforward*. In situations where more implants are used, the degree of implant support increases significantly, in turn increasing the need for well-considered biomechanics and the potential for complications. Thus, these cases are normally considered to be at least *Advanced*.

5.9.3   Loading Protocol

Cochran et al. (2004) concluded that a reasonable amount of evidence exists to support the immediate loading of four rigidly splinted implants with a mandibular overdenture. However, this process is more logistically complex and has a greater risk of complications than the use of early or conventional loading protocols. Thus, any immediate loading procedure would be considered *Complex*.

5.9.4   Esthetic Risk

Generally, mandibular overdentures carry little esthetic risk. However, when the patient's expectations for the esthetic outcome are significant and unlikely to be met using this technique, other treatment options might best be considered. If the overdenture option must be employed, a classification of at least *Advanced* will apply.

5.9.5   Interim Restorations

Mandibular complete dentures often have low levels of retention and stability as a consequence of post-extraction ridge resorption. Implant stabilization and retention of these prostheses have been shown to be related to significant improvements in quality of life. However, during the healing phase after implant placement, these poorly stabilized dentures pose significant risks of uncontrolled loading to the healing implants. It is often better to counsel patients not to wear their lower denture during osseointegration of the dental implants. If denture wear is necessary, higher risks of complications may be expected, and a classification of *Advanced* or higher may be appropriate.

5.9.6   Occlusal Parafunction

As mentioned in 5.8.5, occlusal parafunction will increase the risk of technical complications and the need for maintenance visits (Figure 1). Care should be taken to address this potentially destructive process through a more frequent recall schedule and occlusal equilibration. Consideration should be given to fabrication of a second (back-up) prosthesis to be used in the event that restorative complications arise.

A. Dawson, W. Martin, U. Belser

5.10 Conclusion

The tables and discussion in this chapter detail the issues that have an impact on restorative classification for the case types discussed. Generally, the tables outline the most significant modifying factors influencing the particular case type. The lowest level of complexity defined in these tables can be considered to be the normative classification.

When using these tables to determine the level of classification for a particular case, readers should attempt to match their specific case details to the criteria defined in the appropriate table. The classification that best fits the specific case can then be used in developing a treatment plan for that particular case.

It should be noted that the other modifiers discussed in Chapter 3 may also have an impact on specific cases. Such additional factors will generally act to increase the complexity and/or risk of the process and will likely result in the application of a higher classification than that indicated in the tables being used for that case.

In the following chapter, a number of clinical treatment cases will be discussed in order to illustrate the application of the processes detailed in the preceding parts of this text.

6 Practical Application of the SAC Classification

Having discussed the structure and determinants of the SAC Classification in earlier chapters, in this section the process of determining an SAC Classification for clinical cases will be demonstrated. A number of case presentations will illustrate how a classification may be derived, and some significant issues that may arise.

6.1 How is a Classification Derived for Specific Case?

A. Dawson, S. Chen

During the Mallorca Consensus Conference, the tables that form the basis of discussions in Chapters 4 and 5 were developed. These outline the normative classifications that would be assigned to a class of similar cases, for example, single tooth replacements in an esthetic site. When determining a classification for a specific case within such a class, users of the classification should start by finding the appropriate case type within these tables (for both the surgical and restorative parts of the classification) and deciding on the normative classification that would apply. These surgical and restorative normative classifications can then be further modified to take account of specific risk factors that apply to the case in question to determine the final classification for that case. As esthetic risk is an important part of both the surgical and restorative classification, the ERA (Esthetic Risk Assessment) from Section 3.2 will need to be determined.

The surgical group at the consensus conference proposed six factors that form the basis of their classification. Thus the surgical normative classification can be found by finding the case type and features of the case in question in the tables in Chapter 4. The restorative process is much more complex in the sense that more factors have the potential to influence the outcome of restorative implant treatments. Consequently, the classification for a specific case will be determined by the "best-fit" that can be derived for that case within the appropriate table in Chapter 5. Other potential complicating factors are then applied. In the restorative tables, more than three factors that have an *Advanced* or *Complex* classification would indicate a normative classification of at least *Advanced*. The process might better be described using a number of real-life cases, and these are detailed below.

6.2   A *Straightforward* Restorative Case – Replacement of a Maxillary First Molar

S. Chen, A. Dickinson

A 37-year-old female patient was referred for replacement of an upper right first molar (tooth 16). The pre-treatment status of this area is illustrated in Figure 1. The tooth had been endodontically-treated twice over a 5 year period. Two years previously, the tooth had fractured and was then restored with a post-retained crown. The crown had recently loosened and fallen off.

On examination, the tooth had been decoronated with some post and core structure remaining. Two posts were retaining an amalgam core. A periapical area was present over the mesio-buccal root. Normal probing pockets were present around the tooth. The endodontic and restorative prognosis was deemed to be poor and a replacement with an implant-supported crown was recommended. The remaining dentition was healthy. The patient's general health was good and she was a non-smoker.

The treatment plan was as follows:

1. Extraction of tooth 16, followed by a healing period of 12 weeks to allow partial bone healing and flattening of the sinus floor
2. Implant placement
3. Restoration with a single crown

A surgical SAC assessment was undertaken (Table 1). There were no medical contraindications to treatment and the patient was a non-smoker. The site was not in the esthetic zone. Following extraction of the tooth, it was anticipated that oro-facial bone width would be sufficient to allow an implant with a large endosseous diameter and wide restorative platform to be placed. Bone was expected to reduce in height during the 12 weeks after extraction due to a combination of crestal bone loss and modeling of the bone at the sinus floor. However, it was anticipated that there would be sufficient bone height to allow an 8 mm long implant to be placed. The procedure could therefore be undertaken with minimal anatomic risk. The procedure was determined to have a relatively low level of difficulty, with a low risk of operative and postoperative complications. The surgical SAC Classification was therefore determined to be *Straightforward*.

It was recognized that healing after tooth extraction may result in less bone height than anticipated. In this situation, grafting of the sinus floor using the osteotome technique would be required in conjunction with implant treatment. This procedure would have an increased anatomic risk and complexity. The risk of perforation of the sinus membrane was also recognized.

Significant issues in the determination of a restorative SAC Classification are listed in Table 2. In this case, the space available for restoration was ideal, there was low esthetic risk, and risk of complications was low. As such, all of the applicable factors in Table 2 indicate that a classification of *Straightforward* was appropriate.

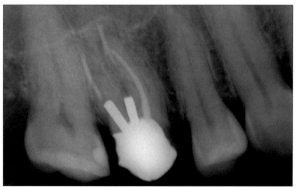

Figure 1.   Radiograph of tooth 16 prior to its final failure.

Table 1. Surgical SAC Classification for the Case of an Upper Molar to be Restored with a Single Implant-Supported Restoration, at initial presentation.

General Factors	Assessment	Notes
Medical contraindications	None	
Smoking habit	None	
Growth considerations	None	
Site Factors	**Assessment**	**Notes**
Bone volume	Sufficient	Possibility that there may not be sufficient bone height following healing after tooth extraction
Anatomic risk	Low	
Esthetic risk	Low	
Complexity	Low	
Risk of complications	Low	Risk of perforation of the sinus floor membrane if site over-drilled
Loading protocol	Early	The plan was to restore the implant 6 to 8 weeks after placement
SAC Classification	Straightforward	

Table 2. Restorative Classification for Implant Replacement of a Single Molar Tooth with a Cemented Restoration.

Posterior Single Tooth	Notes	Straightforward	Advanced	Complex
Inter-arch distance	Refers to the distance from the proposed implant restorative margin to the opposing occlusion	Ideal tooth height +/- 1 mm	Tooth height reduced by ≥ 2 mm	Non-restorable without adjunctive preparatory therapy due to severe over-eruption of opposing dentition
Mesio-distal space (Premolar)		Anatomic space corresponding to the missing tooth +/- 1 mm	Anatomic space corresponding to the missing tooth plus 2 mm or more	Non-restorable without adjunctive preparatory therapy due to severe space restriction ≤ 5 mm
Mesio-distal space (Molar)		Anatomic space corresponding to the missing tooth +/- 1 mm	Anatomic space corresponding to the missing tooth +/- 2 mm or more	Non-restorable without adjunctive preparatory therapy due to severe space restriction ≤ 5 mm
Access		Adequate	Restricted	Access prohibits implant therapy
Loading protocol	To date, immediate restoration and loading procedures are lacking scientific documentation	Conventional or early	Immediate	
Esthetic risk	Refer to ERA (Treatment Guide 1)	Low	Moderate	Maxillary first premolars in patients with high esthetic demands
Occlusal para-function	Risk of complication to the restoration is high	Absent		Present
Provisional implant-supported restorations	Situations where provisional restorations are recommended	Restorative margin < 3 mm apical to mucosal margin	Restorative margin > 3 mm apical to mucosal margin	

The treatment plan was discussed with the patient. The possibility that treatment could increase in complexity if bone height was less than anticipated was highlighted. The patient then gave her consent to proceed with treatment.

The tooth was extracted without flap elevation, and healing progressed uneventfully. After 12 weeks, the soft tissues had healed with minimal loss of oro-facial dimension of the ridge. Radiographically, partial bone fill had oc-curred. However, there was greater vertical loss of bone height than originally anticipated. It was estimated that 6 mm of corono-apical bone was available. It was therefore planned to elevate the floor of the sinus using osteotomes to allow an implant with a length of 8 mm to be placed. The patient was advised that this would increase the degree of difficulty of the procedure, and risk of perforation of the sinus membrane. The SAC Classification was reviewed and amended to *Complex* (Table 3).

Table 3. Surgical SAC Classification for the Case of an Upper Molar to be Restored with a Single Implant-Supported Restoration, after Extraction of the Tooth.

General Factors	Assessment	Notes
Medical contraindications	None	
Smoking habit	None	
Growth considerations	None	
Site Factors	**Assessment**	**Notes**
Bone volume	Insufficient	Sinus floor elevation and bone graft required; sufficient bone height to allow simultaneous implant placement
Anatomic risk	High	Involvement of the maxillary sinus
Esthetic risk	Low	
Complexity	High	Combination of sinus floor elevation using the osteotome technique and implant placement has a high degree of complexity
Risk of complications	High	Risk of perforation of the sinus floor membrane
Loading protocol	Early	The plan was to restore the implant 6 to 8 weeks after placement
SAC Classification	Complex	

Following administration of local anesthesia, full thickness flaps were raised on the facial and palatal aspect of site 16. Intra-operative assessment confirmed sufficient oro-facial bone width to allow an implant with an endosseous diameter of 4.8 mm to be placed. The site was prepared to a depth of 5 mm using twist drills of increasing diameter until the osteotomy was prepared to a diameter of 4.2 mm. The osteotomy was filled with autogenous bone chips that were locally harvested. Osteotomes were used to infracture the cortical bone of the sinus floor. The membrane was checked to verify that no perforation had occurred. An implant with an SLA surface, 4.8 mm endosseous diameter, 8 mm length and 2.8 mm collar (Straumann WN S implant, Straumann AG, Basel, Switzerland) was inserted into the osteotomy. The implant achieved good initial stability and a 2 mm extended healing cap was attached.

The flaps were adapted around the healing cap and closed with simple interrupted sutures. The patient was advised to use a 0.2% chlorhexidine mouth rinse and to refrain from mechanical cleaning of the area for 2 weeks. Healing progressed uneventfully and the implant integrated (Figure 2).

Restorative procedures commenced eight weeks after surgery. This involved the placement of a solid abutment followed by taking a transfer impression that incorporated recording the position of the implant collar and the abutment. At a subsequent appointment, a cemented crown was placed after confirming fit, occlusal and interproximal contacts, and esthetics. The patient was happy with the final result.

At the most recent review, the peri-implant tissues were healthy with stable bone conditions observed nine years after initial surgery (Figures 3a to 3c).

Comments

This case illustrates the surgical and restorative SAC Classifications for replacement of a single upper molar. Initially, the surgical SAC was regarded as *Straightforward*. However following extraction of the tooth, the reduced bone volume increased the complexity of the treatment. This contingency was discussed with the patient before commencement of treatment. The restorative phase of treatment remained *Straightforward* despite the amendment to the surgical classification. The implant was well positioned which allowed restorative treatment to progress as originally planned.

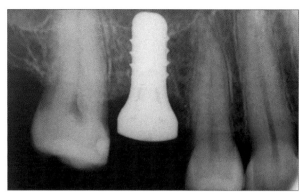

Figure 2.   Radiographic appearance of the healing implant.

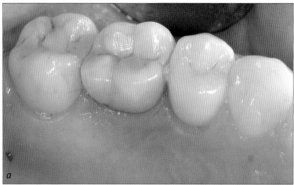

a

Figures 3a-c.   Final restoration in place and radiographic view nine years after surgery.

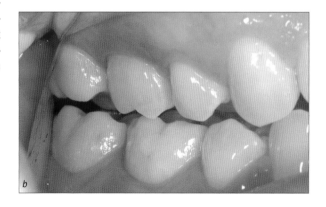

b

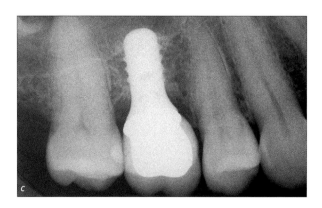

c

6.3 An *Advanced* Case – Upper Left Central Incisor Replacement

C. Evans, S. Chen

A healthy 47-year-old female presented for consultation on referral from her general dental practitioner. The patient had noticed some intermittent bleeding after tooth brushing from the facial surface of the tooth 21. No pain or discomfort had been experienced by the patient. The patient had been referred to a specialist endodontist who confirmed the presence of external cervical resorption (Figure 1). The tooth was deemed not restorable and replacement alternatives sought. The patient wished to investigate the option of an implant-supported crown to replace the upper left central incisor.

Clinical examination revealed tooth 21 to have a small mesial resin restoration but otherwise to be unrestored. Close examination revealed the facial surface of tooth 21 to have a resorptive defect that could be easily probed, extending beneath the gingival margin. The cervical enamel was pink in color indicating the loss in dentinal tooth structure that characterizes these lesions (Figure 2). The adjacent teeth were unrestored. A low smile line was present even on wide smiling. The gingival tissue biotype was classified as medium and the tooth shape was square. Esthetic Risk Assessment indicated that the Esthetic Risk was moderate (Table 1).

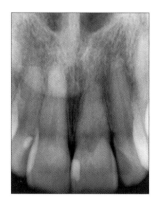

Figure 1. Radiograph of presenting condition of tooth 21.

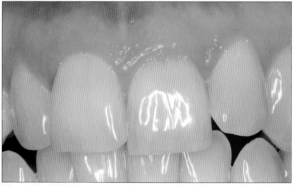

Figure 2. Clinical appearance at presentation, demonstrating pink coloration of the cervical area of tooth 21.

Table 1. Esthetic Risk Assessment.

Esthetic Risk Factor	Level of Risk		
	Low	Moderate	High
Medical status	Healthy, co-operative patient with an intact immune system.		Reduced immune system
Smoking habit	Non-smoker	Light smoker (< 10 cigs/day)	Heavy smoker (> 10 cigs/day)
Patient's esthetic expectations	Low	Medium	High
Lip line	Low	Medium	High
Gingival biotype	Low scalloped, thick	Medium scalloped, medium thick	High scalloped, thin
Shape of tooth crowns	Rectangular		Triangular
Infection at implant site	None	Chronic	Acute
Bone level at adjacent teeth	≤ 5 mm to contact point	5.5 to 6.5 mm to contact point	≥ 7 mm to contact point
Restorative status of neighboring teeth	Virgin		Restored
Width of edentulous span	1 tooth (≥ 7 mm)	1 tooth (≤ 7mm)	2 teeth or more
Soft tissue anatomy	Intact soft tissue		Soft tissue defects
Bone anatomy of alveolar crest	Alveolar crest without bone deficiency	Horizontal bone deficiency	Vertical bone deficiency

There was minimal evidence of parafunctional activity. Tooth 21 had supra-erupted by 0.5 to 1.0 mm compared to the contra-lateral tooth. The gingival margin associated with tooth 21 was irregular and located about 0.5 mm coronal when compared to tooth 11. Crown coloration of the anterior teeth was low in value with strong chroma and a moderate degree of translucency.

Treatment options were discussed with the patient and an implant-supported crown was planned to replace the tooth 21. The case was classified as *Advanced*. An interim removable partial denture was planned to be used during implant therapy.

Due to the intact nature of the root form and lack of apical infection, the surgical phase of implant treatment was planned to be performed as a Type 1 (immediate placement) protocol. Implant placement was planned to allow direct occlusal screw access of the final restoration. A conventional loading protocol was planned with restoration planned after 3 months of implant healing.

The intention to use a Type 1 placement protocol with a flapless approach indicates a surgical SAC Classification of *Complex* (Table 2).

Table 2. Surgical SAC Classification Determination.

General Factors	Assessment	Notes
Medical contraindications	None	
Smoking habit	None	
Growth considerations	None	
Site Factors	**Assessment**	**Notes**
Bone volume	Adequate	
Anatomic risk	Low	
Esthetic risk	Moderate	
Complexity	High	Immediate placement and flapless approach increases complexity of treatment.
Risk of complications	High	
Loading protocol	Conventional	The plan was to restore the implant 12 weeks after placement
SAC Classification	Complex	

The restorative SAC Classification is determined by reference to the relevant case type table (Table 3). This indicates a classification of *Advanced* is warranted. Here, the majority of factors applicable to this case fall into the *Advanced* class, thus indicating this as the appropriate classification.

After minimally traumatic tooth extraction, an implant with an SLA surface (Straumann RN SP implant with an endosseous length of 10 mm, Straumann AG, Basel, Switzerland) was placed in an ideal three dimensional position, to allow direct screw access through the cingulum of the final crown. The implant was placed oro-facially with the shoulder positioned in the *Comfort Zone* as described by Buser et al. 2004. The implant shoulder was located 2.5 mm apical to the planned mucosal margin (Figures 3a and 3b).

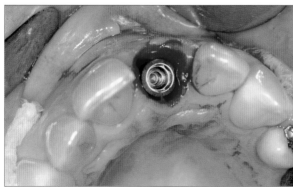 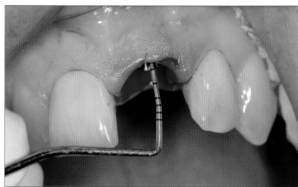

Figures 3a and 3b.   Implant positioning relative to adjacent teeth and the gingival margin.

Table3. Restorative SAC Classification Determination.

Anterior Single Tooth	Notes	Straightforward	Advanced	Complex
Maxillo-mandibular relationship	Refers to horizontal and vertical overlap and the effect on restorability and esthetic outcome	Angle Class I and III	Angle Class II Div 1 and 2	Non-restorable without adjunctive preparatory therapy due to severe malocclusion
Mesio-distal space (maxillary central)	Symmetry is essential for successful outcome		Symmetry +/- 1 mm of contra-lateral tooth	Asymmetry greater than 1 mm
Mesio-distal space (maxillary laterals and canines)		Symmetry +/- 1 mm of contra-lateral tooth	Asymmetry greater than 1 mm	
Mesio-distal space (mandibular anterior)		Symmetry +/- 1 mm of contra-lateral tooth	Asymmetry greater than 1 mm	
Loading protocol	To date, immediate restoration and loading procedures are lacking scientific documentation	Conventional or early		Immediate
Esthetic risk	Refer to ERA (Treatment Guide 1)	Low	Moderate	High
Occlusal para-function	Risk of complication is to the restoration, not to implant survival	Absent		Present
Provisional implant-supported restorations	Provisional restorations are recommended		Restorative margin < 3 mm apical to mucosal margin	Restorative margin > 3 mm apical to mucosal margin

A small connective tissue graft was placed in the facial pouch to augment the facial peri-implant tissue thickness. Implant healing occurred in a partially submerged approach (Figure 4).

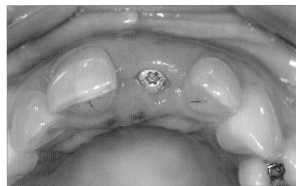

Figure 4.   Implant appearance after completion of healing.

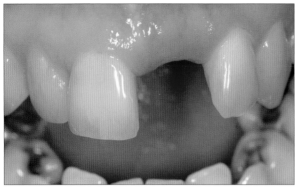

Figure 5.   Soft tissue contour after healing.

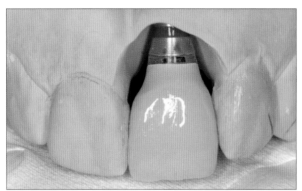

Figure 6.   The completed restoration prior to placement.

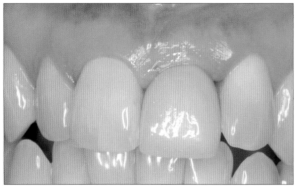

Figure 7.   Final restoration at the time of placement. The emergence profile was modified to minimize soft tissue blanching.

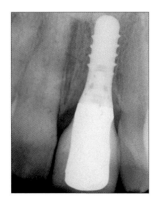

Figure 8.   Radiograph of the seated restoration taken at the time of restoration delivery.

Prior to the commencement of restorative procedures, a second surgical procedure was performed to attach a longer healing abutment to facilitate restorative procedures. An idealized soft tissue form was found with excellent soft tissue contours (Figure 5). The decision was made to proceed direct to definitive restoration, without the need to use a provisional crown to develop the transition zone, due to the ideal implant position, ideal soft tissue volume, low lip line and moderate patient expectations.

Implant restoration was commenced with an implant level impression made to allow fabrication of a master cast. A screw retained impression coping was connected to the implant and a periapical radiograph taken to verify complete seating of the impression coping. A synOcta 1.5mm abutment (Straumann AG, Basel, Switzerland) was selected and a preformed gold coping used to fabricate a direct screw-retained, PFM crown, designed with an idealized emergence profile (Figure 6).

The definitive abutment was tightened to 35 Ncm and retention screw to 15 Ncm. Initial soft tissue blanching required the emergence profile to be reduced slightly to ensure that soft tissue blanching was minimized (Figure 7) and this completely resolved within 10 minutes. Proximal contact points were placed to be within 5 mm of the bone crest level on the adjacent teeth and periapical radiographs demonstrate complete seating of the restoration (Figure 8).

The final restoration required a small amount of surface glaze staining to balance restoration coloration under natural lighting conditions.

The final restoration is seen in harmony with the adjacent teeth and soft tissues 18 months after restoration placement (Figures 9a and 9b).

Comments

This case progressed without any significant complication due to good preoperative assessment and planning, and meticulous execution of the treatment plan by skilled practitioners. However, although this is seemingly a simple case, the inherent risks associated with the procedures used, and the complexity of the techniques employed, still indicate that a surgical classification of *Complex* and a restorative classification of *Advanced* were appropriate.

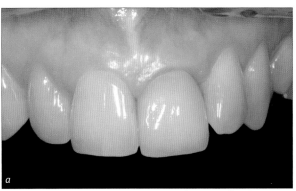

a

Figures 9a and 9b.   *Appearance 18 months after restoration placement.*

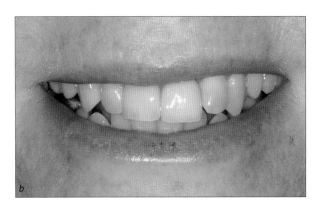

b

6.4   A *Complex* Esthetic Application – Immediate Implant Placement and Provisionalization

F. Higginbottom, T. Wilson

A 35-year-old patient sought help for a failing central incisor. The patient presented with a damaged central incisor that sustained trauma in her teenage years. The root fracture healed with a fibrous union that was stable over time. The restoration eventually failed and definitive treatment plans involved tooth removal and implant placement. The tooth was scheduled for extraction but upon examination it was found that there was a low crest on the facial aspect and the gingival margin at this time was equal with the adjacent central incisor. It was feared that with these findings there would be significant soft tissue change if the tooth were removed. It was decided to orthodontically extrude the tooth and stabilize for one month prior to tooth removal (Figures 1a to 1c). With this procedure the bone and soft tissue relationship was maximized relative to the adjacent tooth.

Risk assessment and pretreatment planning involved determination of ERA and surgical and restorative SAC Classifications. These are illustrated in Tables 1, 2 and 3.

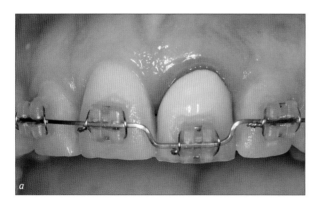

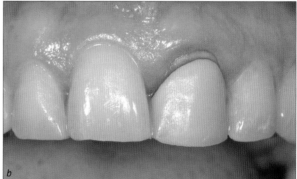

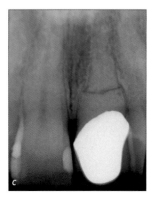

Figures 1a, 1b and 1c.
Orthodontic extrusion of tooth 21 to maximize crestal bone height.

Table 1. Esthetic Risk Assessment.

Esthetic Risk Factor	Level of Risk		
	Low	Moderate	High
Medical status	Healthy, co-operative patient with an intact immune system.		Reduced immune system
Smoking habit	Non-smoker	Light smoker (< 10 cigs/day)	Heavy smoker (> 10 cigs/day)
Patient's esthetic expectations	Low	Medium	High
Lip line	Low	Medium	High
Gingival biotype	Low scalloped, thick	Medium scalloped, medium thick	High scalloped, thin
Shape of tooth crowns	Rectangular		Triangular
Infection at implant site	None	Chronic	Acute
Bone level at adjacent teeth	≤ 5 mm to contact point	5.5 to 6.5 mm to contact point	≥ 7 mm to contact point
Restorative status of neighboring teeth	Virgin		Restored
Width of edentulous span	1 tooth (≥ 7 mm)	1 tooth (≤ 7mm)	2 teeth or more
Soft tissue anatomy	Intact soft tissue		Soft tissue defects
Bone anatomy of alveolar crest	Alveolar crest without bone deficiency	Horizontal bone deficiency	Vertical bone deficiency

Table 2. Surgical SAC Assessment.

General Factors	Assessment	Notes
Medical contraindications	None	
Smoking habit	None	
Growth considerations	None	
Site Factors	**Assessment**	**Notes**
Bone volume	Adequate	
Anatomic risk	Low	
Esthetic risk	Moderate	
Complexity	High	Immediate placement and flapless approach increases treatment complexity.
Risk of complications	High	
Loading protocol	Immediate Restoration	The implant would be subject to some functional loading.
SAC Classification	Complex	

Table 3. Restorative SAC Determination.

Anterior Single Tooth	Notes	Straightforward	Advanced	Complex
Maxillo-mandibular relationship	Refers to horizontal and vertical overlap and the effect on restorability and esthetic outcome	Angle Class I and III	Angle Class II Div 1 and 2	Non-restorable without adjunctive preparatory therapy due to severe malocclusion
Mesio-distal space (maxillary central)	Symmetry is essential for successful outcome		Symmetry +/- 1 mm of contra-lateral tooth	Asymmetry greater than 1 mm
Mesio-distal space (maxillary laterals and canines)		Symmetry +/- 1 mm of contra-lateral tooth	Asymmetry greater than 1 mm	
Mesio-distal space (mandibular anterior)		Symmetry +/- 1 mm of contra-lateral tooth	Asymmetry greater than 1 mm	
Loading protocol	To date, immediate restoration and loading procedures are lacking scientific documentation	Conventional or early		Immediate
Esthetic risk	Refer to ERA (Treatment Guide 1)	Low	Moderate	High
Occlusal para-function	Risk of complication is to the restoration, not to implant survival	Absent		Present
Provisional implant-supported restorations	Provisional restorations are recommended		Restorative margin < 3 mm apical to mucosal margin	Restorative margin > 3 mm apical to mucosal margin

These assessments show that this case had a moderate esthetic risk, and that the SAC Classification from both the surgical and restorative points of view was *Complex*.

The tooth was removed and an implant placed as a Type 1 procedure using a flapless approach (Straumann RN SP implant and SLA surface with a 12 mm endosseous length, Straumann AG, Basel, Switzerland). The implant was placed leaving a horizontal defect dimension. The defect was grafted with hard and soft tissues and enamel matrix derivative (Emdogain™; Straumann AG, Basel, Switzerland) applied. A solid abutment was placed and hand tightened (Figures 2a and 2b). A provisional restoration was placed and left out of functional contact (Figure 2c).

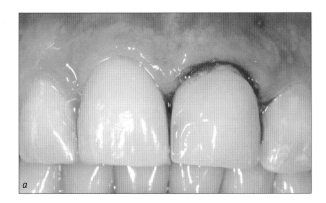

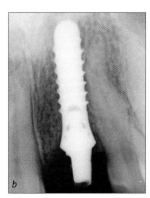

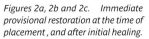

Figures 2a, 2b and 2c.   Immediate provisional restoration at the time of placement , and after initial healing.

The implant was allowed to integrate for twelve weeks. This period proved uneventful. Restorative procedures were commenced with an implant level impression and a new provisional restoration fabricated on a solid abutment (Figures 3a and 3b). The final PFM restoration was fabricated over a synOcta abutment (Straumann AG, Basel, Switzerland) and cast custom mesostructure (Figures 4a and 4b).

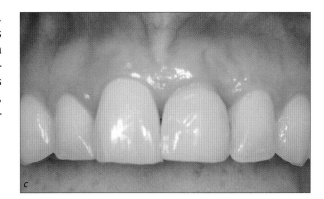

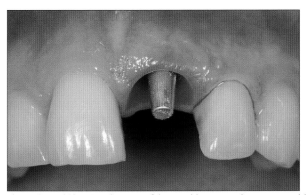

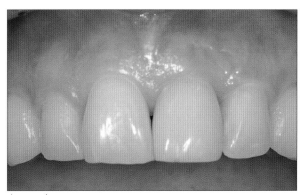

Figures 3a and 3b.   Development of the transition zone using a new provisional restoration.

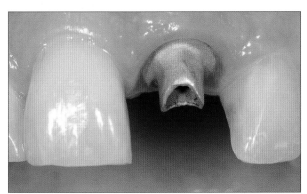

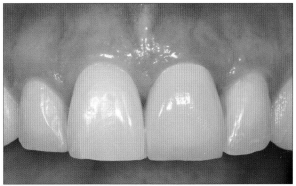

Figures 4a and 4b.   Custom mesostructure and the final cemented crown in place.

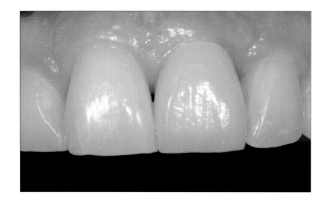

The final result remained stable at the twelve month follow-up appointment (Figures 5a and 5b).

Comments

The techniques employed in this treatment are associated with a high level of complexity and moderate to high risk of complications. Consequently, SAC Classifications of *Complex* are warranted for both the surgical and restorative aspects of treatment. None the less, successful outcomes can be achieved in such cases by careful assessment and patient selection, and through the application of significant skill and experience.

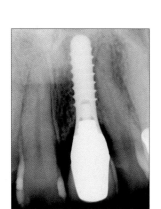

Figures 5a and 5b.   Final result after 12 months in service.

6.5 A Complex Partially Edentulous Case

W. Martin, J. Ruskin

A middle-aged female presented to the clinic with a chief complaint "I am unhappy with my smile and the constant need to remove my teeth at night." The patient was interested in exploring fixed alternatives for restoring her missing anterior teeth.

The patient reported an uncomplicated medical history. She attributed the loss of her anterior teeth to a history of traumatic fractures of teeth 12, 11, 21, and 22. Following the eventual failure of the tooth structure supporting the dental restorations in these sites, extractions were necessary. She presented to the clinic with a RDP replacing the upper incisors that provided adequate functional and esthetic outcomes (Figure 1). The patient presented with a high lip line at full smile.

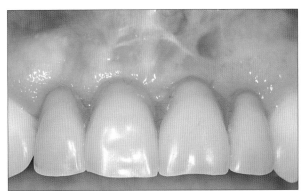

Figure 1. Frontal view with removable dental prosthesis in place.

The patient was free of systemic disease and did not smoke. She reported no history of bruxism or pain related to the temporomandibular joints. A clinical examination of the remaining dentition revealed an occlusal scheme that was within normal limits, a healthy dentition and good periodontal support. Her periodontal home care was excellent with no evidence of plaque or gingivitis. The patient was currently employed in the dental field and educated on dental treatment alternatives, which prompted her to visit our clinic to explore dental implant alternatives.

An evaluation of the anterior edentulous span revealed intra-arch and inter-arch space that was adequate for restoration with four anterior teeth. Her soft tissue height in sites 12 to 22 was coronal to the planned mucosal margins of the proposed restorations, while her ridge width in this area was inadequate to support an ideal emergence profile of these restorations (Figures 2 and 3). A radi-

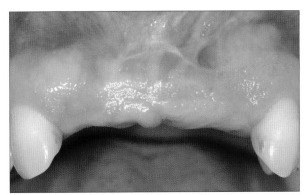

Figure 2. Frontal view of the edentulous space 12 to 22.

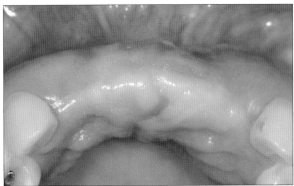

Figure 3. Occlusal view of the edentulous space 12 to 22.

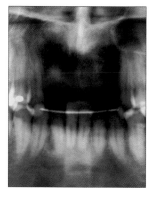

Figure 4.   Isolated panoramic radiograph of the anterior arches.

ographic analysis of this area confirmed the adequate ridge height in the edentulous span and healthy periodontal support of the adjacent teeth 13 and 23 (Figure 4). In the edentulous span, radiolucent areas were located in sites 12 and 22, which were the result of previous root end resection procedures. Tables 1 to 3 highlight the restorative and surgical risk factors associated with this patient's clinical condition.

Table 1: Assessment of Esthetic Risk.

Esthetic Risk Factor	Level of Risk		
	Low	Moderate	High
Medical status	Healthy, co-operative patient with an intact immune system.		Reduced immune system
Smoking habit	Non-smoker	Light smoker (< 10 cigs/day)	Heavy smoker (> 10 cigs/day)
Patient's esthetic expectations	Low	Medium	High
Lip line	Low	Medium	High
Gingival biotype	Low scalloped, thick	Medium scalloped, medium thick	High scalloped, thin
Shape of tooth crowns	Rectangular		Triangular
Infection at implant site	None	Chronic	Acute
Bone level at adjacent teeth	≤ 5 mm to contact point	5.5 to 6.5 mm to contact point	≥ 7 mm to contact point
Restorative status of neighboring teeth	Virgin		Restored
Width of edentulous span	1 tooth (≥ 7 mm)	1 tooth (≤ 7mm)	2 teeth or more
Soft tissue anatomy	Intact soft tissue		Soft tissue defects
Bone anatomy of alveolar crest	Alveolar crest without bone deficiency	Horizontal bone deficiency	Vertical bone deficiency

Table 2: Restorative Risk Factors.

Issue	Degree of Difficulty		
	Low	Moderate	High
Oral Environment			
General Oral Health	No active disease		Active disease
Condition of adjacent teeth	Restored Teeth		Virgin teeth
Reason for tooth loss	Caries/Trauma		Periodontal Disease, or occlusal parafunction
Restorative Volume			
Inter-arch distance	Adequate for planned restoration.	Restricted space, but can be managed.	Adjunctive therapy will be necessary to gain sufficient space for planned restoration.
Mesio-distal space	Sufficient to fit replacements for missing teeth	Some reduction in size, or number of teeth will be necessary	Adjunctive therapy will be needed to achieve a satisfactory result.
Span of restoration	Single tooth	Extended edentulous space	Full arch
Volume and characteristics of the edentulous saddle	No prosthetic soft-tissue replacement will be necessary		Prosthetic replacement of soft tissue will be needed for esthetics or phonetics
Occlusion			
Occlusal Scheme	Anterior guidance		No guidance
Involvement in occlusion	Minimal involvement		Implant restoration is involved in guidance.
Occlusal para-function	Absent		Present
Provisional Restorations			
During implant healing	None required	Removable	Fixed
Implant supported provisionals needed	Not required.	Restorative margin <3mm apical to mucosal crest	Restorative margin >3mm apical to mucosal crest
Loading Protocol	Conventional or early loading		Immediate loading
Materials/Manufacture	Resin based materials ± metal reinforcement	Porcelain fused to metal.	
Maintenance Needs	Low	Moderate	High

Table 3. Surgical SAC Classification.

General Factors	Assessment	Notes
Medical contraindications	None	
Smoking habit	None	
Growth considerations	None	
Site Factors	**Assessment**	**Notes**
Bone volume	Deficient	Horizontal bone augmentation in a staged approachrequired using autologous cortico-cancellous bone block
Anatomic risk	Low	
Esthetic risk	High	As determined by the ERA
Complexity	High	Immediate placement and flapless approach increases treatment complexity.
Risk of complications	High	Implant placement with staged procedures High risk of surgical complications with the bone graft, and donor site morbidity. Complications may significantly affect treatment outcomes
Loading protocol	Conventional or Early	
SAC Classification	Complex	

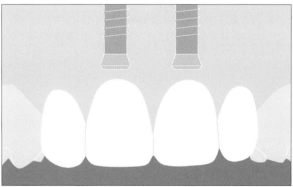

Figure 5.   Dental implants in sites 12 and 22 with a 4-unit fixed dental prosthesis.

The patient was presented with several fixed treatment options. A fixed dental prosthesis supported by teeth 13 and 23 was offered and rejected by the patient due to her unwillingness to have the teeth prepared. Several implant alternatives were proposed, all involving a horizontal ridge augmentation procedure with hard tissue prior to placement of the dental implants. In general, replacement of multiple missing teeth with adjacent implants carries a high esthetic risk due to the inability to control or predict the behavior of the peri-implant tissue (hard and soft) interproximal to the implants. When exploring implant positioning in this region, several alternatives exist, each having carrying strengths and weaknesses (Figures 5 to 7). Lengthy discussions on these risks were covered in detail with the patient at which point she selected the one that allowed her the opportunity for individual teeth. This treatment involved placement of implants in the 12,11,21 and 22 sites. If a treatment of this magnitude was pursued in today's practice, implant designs (bone level implants) that maintain crestal bone while providing enhanced control over emergence profile would be pursued (Figure 8).

The patient's overall proposed treatment was assessed as having a high degree of difficulty and a normative surgical and restorative SAC Classification of *Complex*. When referring to the *Restorative SAC Classification for Anterior Extended Edentulous Spaces*, the patient carried a high esthetic risk while having an ideal intermaxillary relationship with adequate intra-arch space. Several of the modifying factors within this classification carried no added risk to the normal classification other than working with

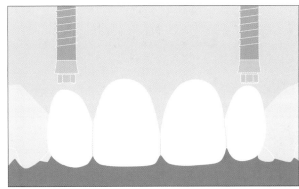

Figure 6.   Dental implants in sites 11 and 21 with a 4-unit fixed dental prosthesis with distal cantilever pontics.

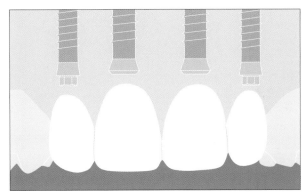

Figure 7.   Dental implants in sites 12, 11, 21 and 22 with four individual implant supported restorations.

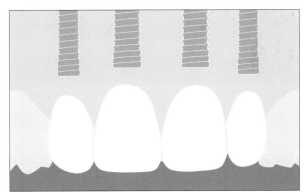

Figure 8.   Bone level dental implants in sites 12, 11, 21 and 22 with four individual implant supported restorations.

Table 4. SAC Decision Matrix for the Maxillary Reconstruction.

Anterior Extended Edentulous Spaces	Notes	Straightforward	Advanced	Complex
Esthetic Risk	Refer for ERA (Treatment Guide 1)	Low	Moderate	High
Intermaxillary relationship	Refers to horizontal and vertical overlap and the effect on restorability and esthetic outcome	Class I and III	Class II Div 1 and 2	Non-restorable without adjunctive preparatory therapy due to severe malocclusion
Mesio-distal space		Adequate for required tooth replacement	Insufficient space available for replacement of all missing teeth	Adjunctive therapy necessary to replace all missing teeth
Occlusion/ Articulation		Harmonious	Irregular with no need for correction	Changes of existing occlusion necessary
Interim restorations during healing		RDP	Fixed	
Provisional implant supported restorations	Provisional restorations are recommended		Restorative margin <3mm apical to mucosal crest	Restorative margin >3mm apical to mucosal crest
Occlusal Para-function	Risk of complication is to the restoration, not implant survival	Absent		Present
Loading protocol	To date immediate restoration and loading procedures are lacking scientific documentation	Conventional or Early		Immediate

implant shoulders that would be located greater than 3mm apical to the mucosal crest (Table 4). The bone volume for implant placement was considered to be inadequate for positioning of the dental implants in an ideal restorative position without the use of a hard tissue augmentation procedure. This type of therapy also carries a moderate classification with consideration to anatomical risk, complexity and risk for complications.

Treatment Phase I: therapy addressing the horizontal ridge deficiency. An onlay graft utilizing an allograft material and resorbable membrane was performed followed by a six-month healing period (Figures 9 and 10). During this healing period an interim removable dental prosthesis was utilized for function and esthetics. Particular attention was given to eliminating any forces on the healing graft site.

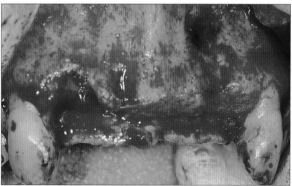

Figure 9.   A frontal view of the ridge deficiency prior to placement of the allogenic graft material.

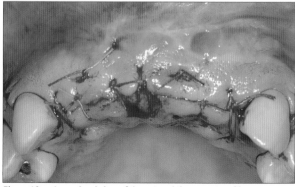

Figure 10.   An occlusal view of the sutured tissue post-grafting.

Treatment Phase II: therapy involved a diagnostic wax-up, template fabrication and positioning of four dental implants in an ideal restoration-driven manner (Figures 11 to 13). The dental implants were placed in a submerged healing protocol in an effort to maximize soft tissue for manipulation during the restorative phase.

Treatment Phase III: during this period the complexity of this treatment became clearly evident. After six weeks of healing, the implants were uncovered with a mid-crestal incision with simultaneous restoration with provisional restorations. Particular attention was given to the inter-proximal contours in an effort to stimulate the formation of papillae. After 8 weeks of healing, deficits in the inter-proximal tissue remained (Figure 14). Periapical radiographs revealed the crestal bone levels adjacent to the implant sites (Figure 15).

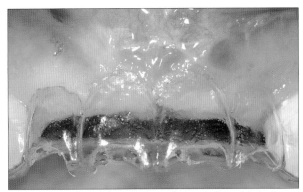

Figure 11. The frontal view with the vertical surgical template in place.

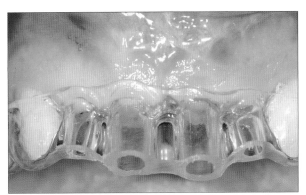

Figure 12. The frontal view with the sleeve surgical template in place.

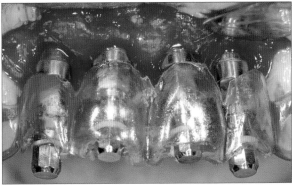

Figure 13. The frontal view of the vertical template highlighting the ideal positioning of the dental implants.

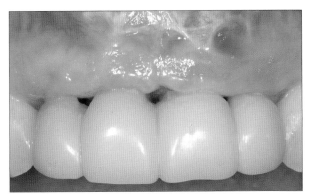

Figure 14. A frontal view of the provisional restorations highlighting the interproximal tissue deficiencies.

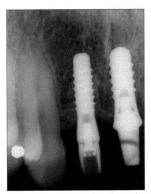
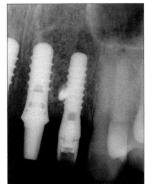

Figure 15. Periapical radiographs of implants in the 12 to 22 sites.

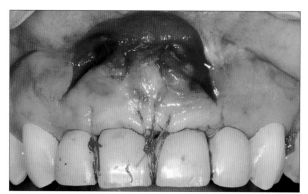

Figure 16.   A post-operative view of the semilunar coronally positioned flap.

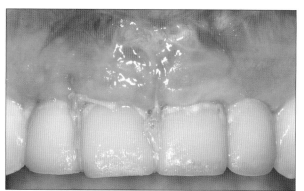

Figure 17.   The frontal view one-week post-surgery.

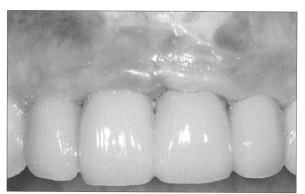

Figure 18.   The frontal view of the provisional restorations post-modification.

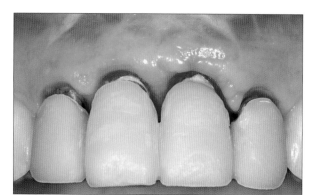

Figure 19.   The frontal view following the gingivoplasty procedure prior to placement of the provisional restorations.

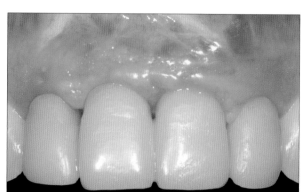

Figure 20.   The frontal view of the provisional restorations after four-weeks of healing.

Careful evaluation of the clinical presentation of the tissue deficiencies compared to the tooth proportions of the provisional restorations prompted us to consider two additional surgical procedures to recover from the esthetic compromise. The first procedure involved a semilunar coronally positioned flap supported by a connective tissue graft. This procedure was performed in an effort to move tissue into areas that would eliminate the interproximal tissue deficits (Figures 16 and 17). Upon healing (4-weeks), the provisional restorations were modified to create ideal emergence profiles (Figure 18).

The provisional restorations were allowed to function for eight-weeks prior to re-evaluation. At the follow-up visit, the patient's smile line and tooth proportions where evaluated and it was determined that longer teeth were necessary to create a harmonious smile line. It should be noted that this finding was due to a successful outcome of the coronally positioned flap procedure. Tissue fill was evident between the implant restorations coronal to the facial surfaces along the mucosal margins. The second surgical procedure would address the mucosal margin positions utilizing surgical gingivoplasty in conjunction with modification of the provisional restorations (Figure 19). After four-weeks of healing, the provisional restorations were re-evaluated and deemed acceptable to proceed with definitive restorations (Figure 20).

Treatment Phase IV: this was initiated with a final impression. Custom abutments utilizing porcelain to create the emergence profile were fabricated in conjunction with all-ceramic zirconia restorations. At delivery, the transition zones created by the provisional restoration can be appreciated (Figure 21). The custom abutments were tightened to 35Ncm and sealed with cotton and cavit (3M ESPE, St. Paul, MN, USA). The restorations were cemented with a definitive resin-modified cement (Figures 22 and 23). The six-month follow-up visit highlights the tissue contours and acceptable esthetic result (Figures 24 to 27).

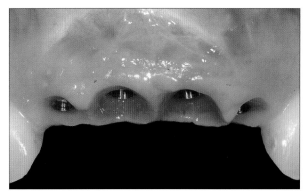

Figure 21.   The frontal view of the transition zone around implants in the 12 – 22 positions.

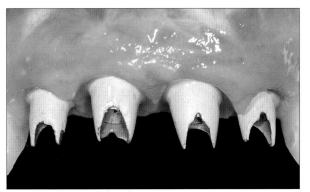

Figure 22.   The frontal view of the custom abutments.

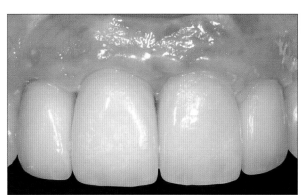

Figure 23.   The frontal view of the implant restorations at delivery.

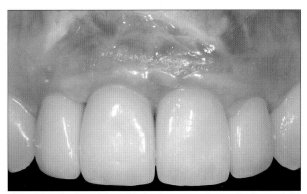

Figure 24.   The frontal view of the implant restorations at the six-month follow-up visit.

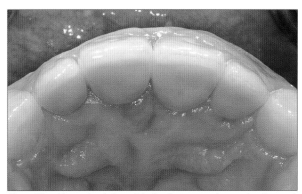

Figure 25.   The occlusal view of the implant restorations at the six-month follow-up visit.

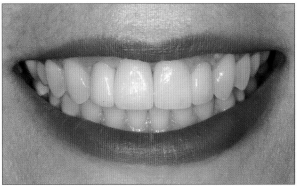

Figure 26.   The patient's smile at the six-month follow-up visit.

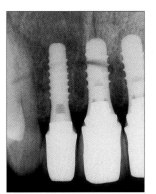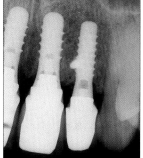

Figure 27.   Periapical radiographs at the six-month follow-up visit.

The authors wish to acknowledge the participation of Dr. N. DeTure and Mr. M. Jim in the treatment team for this case, and to thank them for their significant contribution to the successful outcome.

Comments

This treatment highlighted the complexity of the diagnosis and planning of a patient with high esthetic demands coupled with a difficult clinical situation. Despite the meticulous planning, surgical and restorative treatment procedures, alterations in the planned treatment were required to achieve clinician and patient satisfaction. These alterations mostly resulted from conditions that arose from outcomes of procedures performed during the therapy. While the SAC Classification Tables for this treatment assisted in establishing the initial complexity of this treatment, it should be understood that implant therapy is an evolving process that will require re-assessment of treatment complexity throughout care. This case is a good example of a situation where the final outcome is dependent on the degree of success of intermediary steps which cannot readily be predicted in the treatment planning phase. Such cases warrant classifications of *Complex* because of this uncertainty, as well as the complexity of the treatments used and the risks of complications.

6.6 A Complex Edentulous Case

D. Morton, Z. Rashid, A. Boeckler, H. Hayashi

An elderly gentleman presented complaining of tooth mobility and pain. Additionally, he was concerned with deteriorating esthetics and compromised masticatory function. The patient reported an uncomplicated medical history. He attributed his dental condition to poor professional dental care in his native country, and less than optimal oral hygiene. He was partially dentate (Figures 1a to 1e), his remaining dentition displaying occlusal plane disharmony, drifting and dental caries. His plaque control was historically poor, and he displayed chronic advanced periodontitis. He was able to tolerate removable partial prostheses only on an intermittent basis. Radiographic examination confirmed advanced bone loss and the poor condition of the remaining teeth (Figure 2).

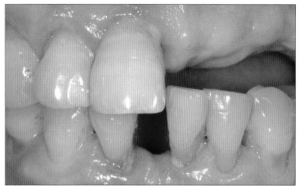

Figure 1a.   Pretreatment view – anterior aspect.

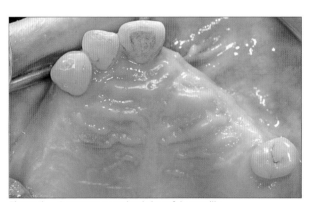

Figure 1b.   Pretreatment occlusal view of the maxilla.

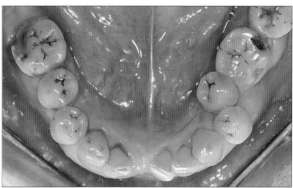

Figure 1c.   Pretreatment occlusal view of the mandible.

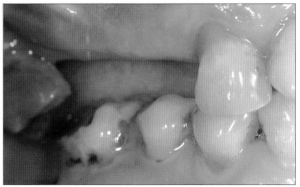

Figure 1d.   Pretreatment right lateral view.

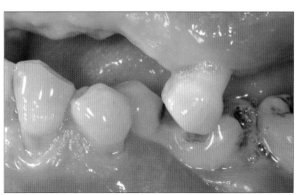

Figure 1e.   Pretreatment left lateral view.

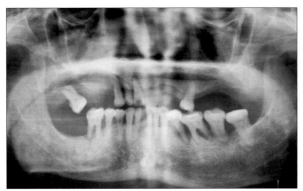

Figure 2.   Pretreatment orthopantomograph.

The patient was free of systemic disease and did not smoke. He was a bruxer, though he suffered no pain in the facial musculature or temporomandibular joints. His chief complaints were tooth pain and mobility, and aesthetic and functional compromise. His treatment expectations were realistic.

The patient was provided with several treatment options. These included definitive complete removable prostheses, implant retained overdentures, and fixed metal-acrylic prostheses. As a result of his limited satisfaction with removable options, the patient elected to proceed with treatment that provided fixed prostheses.

The first phase of treatment involved extraction of the remaining teeth and fabrication of interim maxillary and mandibular complete removable prostheses. The hard and soft tissues were allowed to heal for four months prior to implant placement. Throughout the healing period the patient confirmed his dissatisfaction with the removable prostheses, and complained of limited rest space. A summary of the patient's risk analysis is provided (Tables 1 to 5).

Table 1. Assessment of Esthetic Risk.

Esthetic Risk Factor	Level of Risk		
	Low	Moderate	High
Medical status	Healthy, co-operative patient with an intact immune system.		Reduced immune system
Smoking habit	Non-smoker	Light smoker (< 10 cigs/day)	Heavy smoker (> 10 cigs/day)
Patient's esthetic expectations	Low	Medium	High
Lip line	Low	Medium	High
Gingival biotype	Low scalloped, thick	Medium scalloped, medium thick	High scalloped, thin
Shape of tooth crowns	Rectangular		Triangular
Infection at implant site	None	Chronic	Acute
Bone level at adjacent teeth	≤ 5 mm to contact point	5.5 to 6.5 mm to contact point	≥ 7 mm to contact point
Restorative status of neighboring teeth	Virgin		Restored
Width of edentulous span	1 tooth (≥ 7 mm)	1 tooth (≤ 7mm)	2 teeth or more
Soft tissue anatomy	Intact soft tissue		Soft tissue defects
Bone anatomy of alveolar crest	Alveolar crest without bone deficiency	Horizontal bone deficiency	Vertical bone deficiency

Table 2. Surgical SAC Assessment.

General Factors	Assessment	Notes
Medical contraindications	None	
Smoking habit	None	
Growth considerations	None	
Site Factors	**Assessment**	**Notes**
Bone volume	Sufficient	
Anatomic risk	High	Involvement of the maxillary sinus and/or inferior dental nerve.
Esthetic risk	Moderate	
Complexity	High	Combination of sinus floor elevation using the osteotome technique and implant placement has a high degree of complexity
Risk of complications	High	Risk of perforation of the sinus floor membrane
Loading protocol	Early	The plan was to restore the implant 6 to 8 weeks after placement
SAC Classification	Complex	

Table 3. Restorative Risk Factors.

Issue	Degree of Difficulty		
	Low	Moderate	High
Oral Environment			
General Oral Health	No active disease		Active disease
Condition of adjacent teeth	Restored Teeth		
Reason for tooth loss	Caries/Trauma		Periodontal Disease, or occlusal parafunction
Restorative Volume			
Inter-arch distance	Adequate for planned restoration.	Restricted space, but can be managed.	Adjunctive therapy will be necessary to gain sufficient space for planned restoration.
Mesio-distal space	Sufficient to fit replacements for missing teeth	Some reduction in size, or number of teeth will be necessary	Adjunctive therapy will be needed to achieve a satisfactory result.
Span of restoration	Single tooth	Extended edentulous space	Full arch
Volume and characteristics of the edentulous saddle	No prosthetic soft-tissue replacement will be necessary		Prosthetic replacement of soft tissue will be needed for esthetics or phonetics
Occlusion			
Occlusal Scheme	Anterior guidance		No guidance
Involvement in occlusion	Minimal involvement		Implant restoration is involved in guidance.
Occlusal para-function	Absent		Present
Provisional Restorations			
During implant healing	None required	Removable	Fixed
Implant supported provisionals needed	Not required.	Restorative margin <3mm apical to mucosal crest	Restorative margin >3mm apical to mucosal crest
Loading Protocol	Conventional or early loading		Immediate loading
Materials/Manufacture	Resin based materials ± metal reinforcement	Porcelain fused to metal.	
Maintenance Needs	Low	Moderate	High

Table 4. SAC Decision Matrix for the Maxillary Rehabilitation.

Edentulous Maxilla - Fixed	Notes	Straightforward	Advanced	Complex
Inter-arch distance	Refers to the distance from proposed implant restorative margin to opposing occlusion. Note: hybrid bridge restorations will need more space		Average	Space restricted for adequate restoration.
Access			Good	Restricted
Loading protocol	To date immediate restoration and loading procedures are lacking scientific documentation		Conventional or Early	Immediate
Esthetic Risk	Refer for ERA (Treatment Guide 1)		Low	Moderate/High
Provisional restorations during healing			Removable	Fixed
Occlusal Para-function	Risk of complication is to the restoration, not implant survival		Absent	Present
Occlusal Scheme/ Issues			Anterior Guidance	No Anterior Guidance

Table 5. SAC Decision Matrix for the Mandibular Reconstruction.

Edentulous Mandible - Fixed	Notes	Straightforward	Advanced	Complex
Inter-arch distance	Refers to the distance from proposed implant restorative margin to opposing occlusion. Note: hybrid bridge restorations will need more space		Average	Excessive (Mechanical leverage issues) or restricted (space for components)
Loading protocol	To date immediate restoration and loading procedures are lacking scientific documentation		Conventional or Early	Immediate
Esthetic Risk	Refer for ERA (Treatment Guide 1)		Low	Moderate/High
Provisional restorations during healing			Removable	Fixed
Occlusal Para-function	Risk of complication is to the restoration, not implant survival		Absent	Present
Occlusal Scheme/ Issues			Anterior Guidance	No Anterior Guidance

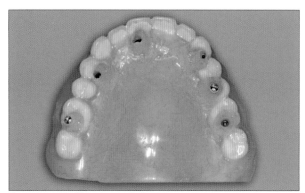

Figure 3a.   Maxillary denture index.

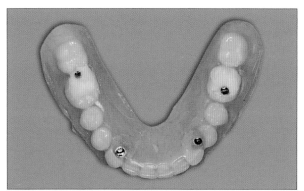

Figure 3b.   Mandibular denture index.

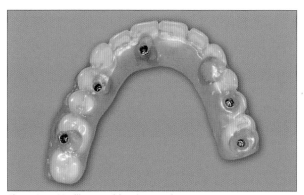

Figure 4a.   Maxillary provisional restoration.

SAC Classification

The patient's overall proposed treatment was assessed as having a high degree of difficulty and a surgical and restorative SAC Classification of *Complex*. The bone volume for implant placement was considered adequate in both arches. However, the plan for fixed treatment of complete arches, particularly the maxilla, was consistent with a surgical classification of *Complex*. The necessity for implant positioning congruent with the proposed teeth, and the concerns relating to inter-arch space were of particular concern.

The intricacy of complete arch prostheses from a clinical and technical perspective is consistent with a *Complex* restorative classification. Additional concerns related to the patient's bruxism habit and the ability of the proposed definitive prostheses to withstand the likely intra-oral forces. The restricted space available for restorative materials and the probability of limitations in the patient's ability to maintain his prostheses were additional likely complications. The patient's restorative classification was therefore considered *Complex*.

The implants were positioned according to templates fabricated as duplicates of his treatment prostheses. To trial his ability to tolerate fixed restorations his existing prostheses were used to index implant position (Figures 3a and 3b), and then modified to provide fixed acrylic resin provisional restorations (Figures 4a to 4c). The fixed provisional restorations allowed the clinicians and the patient to assess the proposed aesthetic and functional outcomes. Complications included the limited inter-arch space and the ability of the patient to maintain the prostheses.

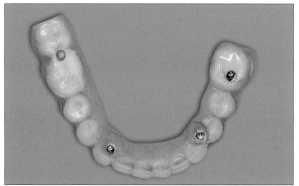

Figure 4b.   Mandibular provisional restoration.

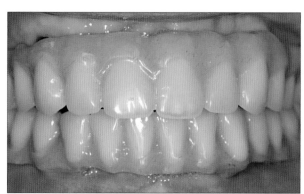

Figure 4c.   Anterior View. Fixed provisional restorations.

Definitive Treatment

Although concerns remained regarding the achievability of an optimal outcome, definitive metal acrylic resin fixed prostheses were fabricated. Implant level impressions were made utilizing impression caps and synOcta positioning cylinders (Straumann AG, Basel, Switzerland) (Figures 5a and 5b). Casts were poured in Type IV dental stone and articulated. A trial set-up was brought to the patient to confirm the proposed vertical dimension of occlusion and aesthetic arrangement (Figure 6).

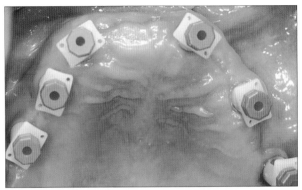

Figure 5a.   Maxillary arch.

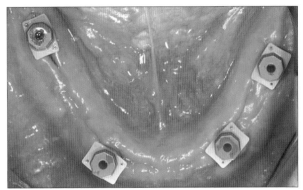

Figure 5b.   Mandibular arch.

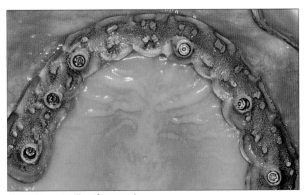

Subsequent to patient acceptance of the trial set-up, frameworks were fabricated and brought to the patient for evaluation of fit (Figures 7a and 7b).

Figure 6.   Anterior view of the trial set-up.

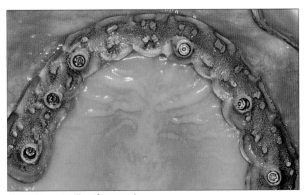

Figure 7a.   Maxillary framework.

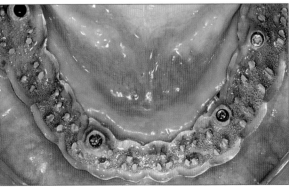

Figure 7b.   Mandibular framework.

Despite efforts to the contrary, the intaglio of both maxillary and mandibular frameworks displayed concavities (Figures 8a and 8b). These were the result of the limited interarch space, and the patient was advised of the maintenance compromise.

The final prostheses were then fabricated by attaching the artificial teeth to the framework with acrylic resin. The patient was initially satisfied with both the aesthetic and functional outcome (Figures 9a to 9d).

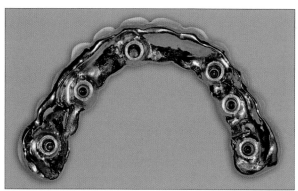

Figure 8a.   Maxillary intaglio.

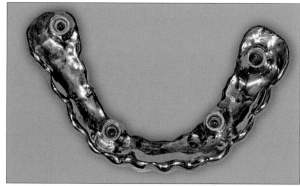

Figure 8b.   Mandibular intaglio.

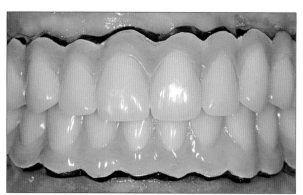

Figure 9a.   Definitive metal acrylic prostheses.

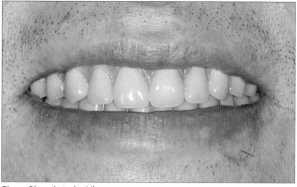

Figure 9b.   Anterior View.

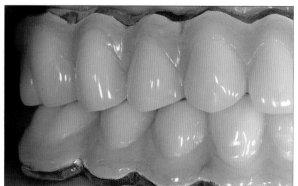

Figure 9c.   Right Lateral View.

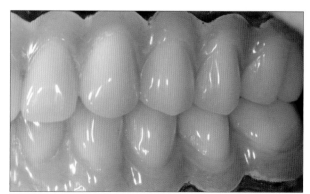

Figure 9d.   Left Lateral View.

In the months following prostheses delivery several complications developed. These included fractured prosthetic teeth, difficulty in oral hygiene maintenance, and an uncomfortable feeling resulting from the restriction in inter-occlusal rest space. Although anticipated, and managed, the complications were numerous and frustrating to both the patient and clinicians.

Such complications are not uncommon with rehabilitations of this type. Space is required not only for aesthetic and functional tooth replacements, but also for metal frameworks of adequate dimension, and acrylic retaining resin. Subsequent to detailed discussions with the patient, replacement of the existing prostheses with metal ceramic alternatives was considered appropriate.

These restorations require less space, and it was felt the patient would be provided with greater comfort through the reduction in vertical dimension, and the recapturing of rest space. Further, the metal frameworks could be extended to include the occlusal surfaces of the posterior teeth, increasing both strength and durability, and further improving the inter-maxillary relationships. Lastly, oral hygiene maintenance was more favorable as a result of the incorporation of modified ridge-lap pontic design, and reduction in ridge-lap.

The proposed aesthetic arrangement was again trialed in acrylic resin to confirm the patient's satisfaction (Figure 10). Casts of the individual interim prostheses were made and cross-articulated with the master casts of each arch.

Plastic abutment replicas were positioned on the maxillary master cast to ensure appropriate inclination for the fabrication of a screw-retained prosthesis. The applicability of the abutments was confirmed using a vacuum formed matrix fabricated on the cast of the provisional restoration (Figures 11a and 11b).

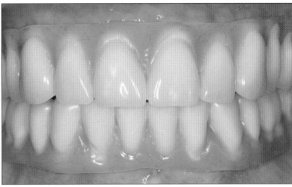

Figure 10. Anterior view of the trial arrangement.

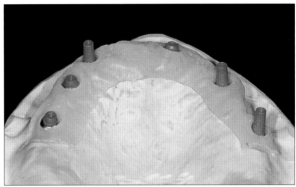

Figure 11a. Plastic abutment replicas.

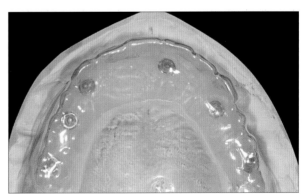

Figure 11b. Vacuum formed matrix.

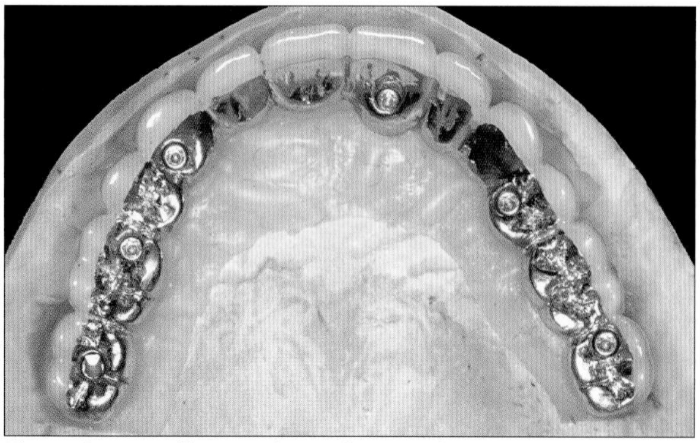

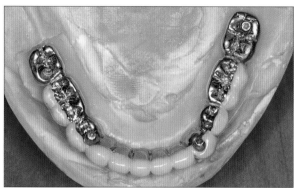

Figure 12a.   Maxillary metal ceramic restoration.

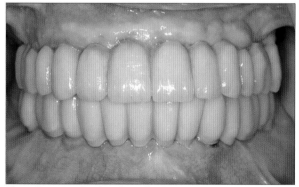

Figure 12b.   Mandibular metal ceramic restoration.

The definitive metal-ceramic restorations were then fabricated. The emergence profile of the prostheses was considered appropriate and capable of being maintained. Occlusal views of the prostheses illustrate the metal occlusal surface, desirable from the perspective of space and durability (Figures 12a and 12b). Ceramic coverage of the buccal cusps of all teeth preserved the aesthetic outcome (Figures 13a and 13b). The patient was provided with an occlusal splint in an effort to reduce the destructive nature of his parafunctional habits.

The patient has now been in non-complicated follow-up for greater than twelve months. The metal-ceramic prostheses have proven durable to date. He has an improved capacity to maintain his prostheses, and is happy from both esthetic and comfort perspectives. Radiographic analysis after twelve months with the metal-ceramic prostheses confirms the health and integrity of the implants and the fit and form of the prostheses (Figure 14).

Surgical Procedures - Dr. J. Green. Director, Oral and Maxillofacial Residency Program. University of Florida Department of Oral and Maxillofacial Surgery and Diagnostic Sciences.

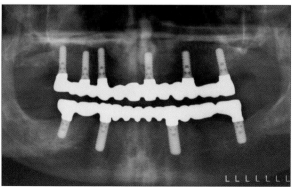

Figure 13a.   Anterior view of completed case.

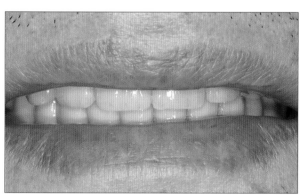

Figure 13b.   Anterior profile of completed case.

Comments

Treatment of this patient was difficult, and despite meticulous planning, treatment alterations were required throughout care. These mostly resulted from conditions diagnosed during assessment and planning. It should be noted that treatment of patients in the *Complex* category increases the likelihood of less than optimal outcomes, and the need for treatment modifications.

Figure 14.   Orthopantomograph one year after prostheses insertion.

6.7 Conclusion

The cases in this chapter illustrate the application of the SAC Classification to the practice of dental implantology. Examples have demonstrated the flexibility of the classification, and its ability to evolve through treatment to adapt to changed circumstances.

The SAC Classification is a useful tool to assist implant dentists of all levels of experience in case selection and treatment planning. It is not, however, infallible, nor is it a replacement for careful assessment and treatment planning, but rather a framework that enhances both of these activities. Additionally, the classification is also a useful shorthand for documenting clinical assessments and for communicating these to other practitioners who are familiar with its structure.

7 <u>Conclusion</u>

A. Dawson, S. Chen

The outcome of dental implant treatment is influenced by four inter-related factors (Figure 1) – the patient, the clinician, the biomaterials used, and the treatment approach (Buser and Chen 2008). In this regard, the clinician's role is central to achieving predictable outcomes whilst minimizing risk to the patient. At the outset, the clinician is responsible for assessing and diagnosing the patient's clinical condition and suitability for treatment. The clinician must then select the most appropriate biomaterials to use and recommend the most appropriate treatment approach. Finally, the clinician must perform the treatment to an appropriate standard of care. Information provided to the patient should include the degree of difficulty of the planned treatment. It is recommended that the SAC Classification be adopted for this purpose.

To assist clinicians in applying the SAC Classification in clinical practice, normative classifications have been given for generic case types. These may then be modified by individual factors specific to the clinical case in question. The SAC Classification is a dynamic tool that can be varied to meet changed circumstances during the course of treatment.

The SAC Classification may assist clinicians on a number of levels. It can provide a framework for documentation of the degree of difficulty and risks involved. This information may be communicated with patients and form the basis for obtaining informed consent. For the novice implant practitioner, the classification assists with selection of cases that are consistent with clinical experience and ability. For more experienced clinicians, the classification can serve as a check-list to assist in risk identification and management.

Finally, the SAC Classification is sufficiently robust in its structure to allow it to adapt as the evidence base, and the techniques and technologies of implant dentistry evolve. The structure and rules will allow the SAC Classification to grow along with implant dentistry, thereby facilitating clinicians, educators and patients into the future.

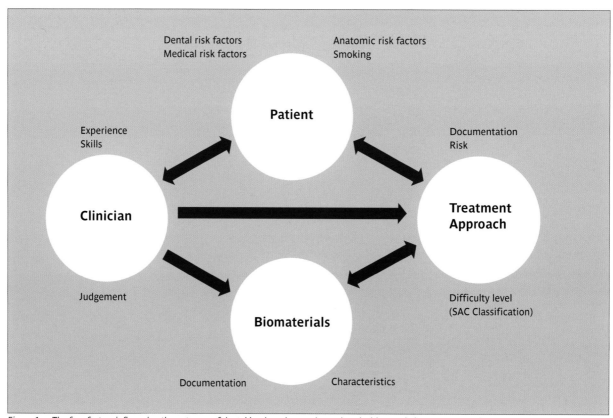

Figure 1.   The four factors influencing the outcome of dental implant therapy (reproduced with permission; Buser and Chen 2008)

8 <u>References</u>

Baelum, V. and Ellegaard, B. (2004) Implant survival in periodontally compromised patients. J Periodontol 75: 1404 – 12.

Behrents, R. G. (1985) Growth in the aging craniofacial skeleton. In Craniofacial growth series; monograph 17, pp. 69 – 128. Ann Arbor, Mich.: University of Michigan.

Belser, U., Buser, D. and Higginbottom, F. (2004) Consensus statements and recommended clinical procedures regarding esthetics in implant dentistry. Int J Oral Maxillofac Implants 19 Suppl: 73 – 4.

Belser, U., Buser, D., Hess, D., Schmid, B., Bernard, J. P. and Lang, N. P. (1998) Aesthetic implant restorations in partially edentulous patients – a critical appraisal. Periodontol 2000 17: 132 – 50.

Block, M. S. and Kent, J. N. (1990) Factors associated with soft and hard tissue compromise of endosseous implants. J Oral Maxillofac Surg 48: 1153 – 60.

Botticelli, D., Berglundh, T. and Lindhe, J. (2004) Hard tissue alterations following immediate implant placement in extraction sites. J Clin Periodontol 31: 820 – 28.

Brägger, U., Aeschlimann, S., Burgin, W., Hämmerle, C. H. and Lang, N. P. (2001) Biological and technical complications and failures with fixed partial dentures (FPD) on implants and teeth after four to five years of function. Clin Oral Implants Res 12: 26 – 34.

Bridger, D. V. and Nicholls, J. I. (1981) Distortion of ceramometal fixed partial dentures during the firing cycle. J Prosthet Dent 45: 507 – 14.

Berglundh T., Persson L. and Klinge B. (2002) A systematic review of the incidence of biological and technical complications in implant dentistry reported in prospective longitudinal studies of at least 5 years. J Clin Periodontol. 29 Suppl 3:197-212.

Buser D. and Chen S. (2008). Factors influencing the treatment outcomes of implants in post-extraction sites. In: ITI Treatment Guide Vol. 3: Implant placement in post-extraction sites. Treatment options, eds. D. Buser et al., pp 18 – 28. Berlin: Quintessence Publishing Co., Ltd.

Buser, D., Martin, W. and Belser, U. C. (2004) Optimizing esthetics for implant restorations in the anterior maxilla: anatomic and surgical considerations. Int J Oral Maxillofac Implants 19 Suppl: 43 – 61.

Buser, D., von Arx, T., ten Bruggenkate, C. and Weingart, D. (2000) Basic surgical principles with ITI implants. Clin Oral Implants Res 11 Suppl 1:59 – 68.

Buser, D. and von Arx, T. (2000) Surgical procedures in partially edentulous patients with ITI implants. Clin Oral Implants Res 11 Suppl: 83 – 100.

Chen S. and Buser D. (2008). Implants in post-extractions sites – A literature update. In: ITI Treatment Guide Vol. 3: Implant placement in post-extraction sites. Treatment options, eds. D. Buser et al., pp 18 – 28. Berlin: Quintessence Publishing Co., Ltd.

Chen, S., Darby, I. B. and Reynolds, E. C. (2007) A prospective clinical study of non-submerged immediate implants: clinical outcomes and esthetic results. Clin Oral Implants Res 18: 552 – 62.

Choquet, V., Hermans, M., Adriaenssens, P., Daelemans, P., Tarnow, D. P. and Malevez, C. (2001) Clinical and radiographic evaluation of the papilla level adjacent to single-tooth dental implants. A retrospective study in the maxillary anterior region. J Periodontol 72: 1364 – 71.

Cochran, D. L., Morton, D. and Weber, H. P. (2004) Consensus statements and recommended clinical procedures regarding loading protocols for endosseous dental implants. Int J Oral Maxillofac Implants 19 Suppl: 109 – 13.

Evans, C. J. D. and Chen, S. T. (2008) Esthetic outcomes of immediate implant placements. Clin Oral Implants Res 19:73 – 80.

Feine, J. S., Carlsson, G. E., Awad, M. A., Chehade, A., Duncan, W. J., Gizani, S., Head, T., Lund, J. P., MacEntee, M., Mericske-Stern, R., Mojon, P., Morais, J., Naert, I., Payne, A. G., Penrod, J., Stoker, G. T., Tawse-Smith, A., Taylor, T. D., Thomason, J. M., Thomson, W. M. and Wismeijer, D. (2002) The McGill consensus statement on overdentures. Mandibular two-implant overdentures as first choice standard of care for edentulous patients. Montreal, Quebec, May 24 – 25, 2002. Int J Oral Maxillofac Implants 17: 601 – 2.

Ferreira, S. D., Silva, G. L., Cortelli, J. R., Costa, J. E. and Costa, F. O. (2006) Prevalence and risk variables for peri-implant disease in Brazilian subjects. J Clin Periodontol 33: 929 – 35.

Fugazzotto, P. A. (2002) Implant placement in maxillary first premolar fresh extraction sockets: description of technique and report of preliminary results. J Periodontol 73: 669 – 74.

Fugazzotto, P. A. (2006) Implant placement at the time of maxillary molar extraction: technique and report of preliminary results of 83 sites. J Periodontol 77: 302 – 9.

Hämmerle C. H., Chen S. T. and Wilson T. G. (2004) Consensus statements and recommended clinical procedures regarding the placement of implants in extraction sockets. Int J Oral Maxillofac Implants 19 Suppl: 26 – 8.

Ibañez J. C., Tahhan M. J., Zamar J. A., Menendez A. B., Juaneda A. M., Zamar N. J. and Monqaut J. L. (2005) Immediate occlusal loading of double acid-etched surface titanium implants in 41 consecutive full-arch cases in the mandible and maxilla: 6- to 74-month results. J Periodontol. 76:1972 – 81.

Johansson, G., Palmqvist, S. and Svenson, B. (1994) Effects of early placement of a single tooth implant. A case report. Clin Oral Implants Res 5: 48 – 51.

Kan, J. Y., Rungcharassaeng, K., Umezu, K. and Kois, J. C. (2003) Dimensions of peri-implant mucosa: an evaluation of maxillary anterior single implants in humans. J Periodontol 74: 557 – 62.

Karl M., Wichmann M. G., Winter W., Graef F., Taylor T. D. and Heckmann S. M. (2008) Influence of fixation mode and superstructure span upon strain development of implant fixed partial dentures. J Prosthodont. 17:3 – 8.

Karoussis, I. K., Salvi, G. E., Heitz-Mayfield, L. J., Brägger, U., Hämmerle, C. H. and Lang, N. P. (2003) Long-term implant prognosis in patients with and without a history of chronic periodontitis: a 10-year prospective cohort study of the ITI Dental Implant System. Clin Oral Implants Res 14: 329 – 39.

Keith S. E., Miller B. H., Woody R. D. and Higginbotton F. L. (1999) Marginal discrepancy of screw-retained and cemented metal-ceramic crowns on implant abutments. Int J Oral Maxillofac Implants 14:369 – 78.

Koch, G., Bergendal, T., Kvint, S. and Johansson, U. B. (1996) Consensus conference on oral implants in young patients. Graphic Systems, Gothenburg, Sweden.

Kois, J. C. (2001) Predictable single tooth peri-implant esthetics: five diagnostic keys. Compend Contin Educ Dent 22: 199 – 206; quiz 208.

Martin, W. C., Morton, D. and Buser, D. (2007) Diagnostic factors for esthetic risk assessment. In ITI Treatment Guide Vol 1: Implant therapy in the esthetic zone - single-tooth replacements, eds. D. Buser et al., pp. 11 – 20. Berlin: Quintessence Publishing Co., Ltd.

Moy, P. K., Medina, D., Shetty, V. and Aghaloo, T. L. (2005) Dental implant failure rates and associated risk factors. Int J Oral Maxillofac Implants 20: 569 – 77.

Müller, H. P. and Eger, T. (1997) Gingival phenotypes in young male adults. J Clin Periodontol 24: 65 – 71.

Oesterle, L. J. and Cronin, R. J., Jr. (2000) Adult growth, aging, and the single-tooth implant. Int J Oral Maxillofac Implants 15: 252 – 60.

Oesterle, L. J., Cronin, R. J., Jr. and Ranly, D. M. (1993) Maxillary implants and the growing patient. Int J Oral Maxillofac Implants 8: 377 – 87.

Olsson, M., Lindhe, J. and Marinello, C. P. (1993) On the relationship between crown form and clinical features of the gingiva in adolescents. J Clin Periodontol 20: 570 – 7.

Op Heij, D. G., Opdebeeck, H., van Steenberghe, D., Kokich, V. G., Belser, U. and Quirynen, M. (2006) Facial development, continuous tooth eruption, and mesial drift as compromising factors for implant placement. Int J Oral Maxillofac Implants 21: 867 – 78.

Op Heij, D. G., Opdebeeck, H., van Steenberghe, D. and Quirynen, M. (2003) Age as compromising factor for implant insertion. Periodontol 2000 33: 172 – 84.

Ortorp A. and Jemt, T. (2006) Clinical experiences with laser-welded titanium frameworks supported by implants in the edentulous mandible: a 10-year follow-up study. Clin Implant Dent Relat Res 8:198 – 209.

Paolantonio, M., Dolci, M., Scarano, A., d'Archivio, D., di Placido, G., Tumini, V. and Piattelli, A. (2001) Immediate implantation in fresh extraction sockets. A controlled clinical and histological study in man. J Periodontol 72: 1560 – 71.

Sailer, H. F. and Pajarola, G. F. (1999) Oral surgery for the general dentist., Stuttgart, Thieme Medical Publishers.

Schropp, L., Wenzel, A., Kostopolous, L. and Karring, T. (2003) Bone healing and soft tissue contour changes following single-tooth extraction: A clinical and radiographic 12-month prospective study. Int J Periodont Rest Dent 23: 313 – 23.

Strietzel, F. P., Reichart, P. A., Kale, A., Kulkarni, M., Wegner, B. and Kuchler, I. (2007) Smoking interferes with the prognosis of dental implant treatment: a systematic review and meta-analysis. J Clin Periodontol 34: 523 – 44.

Summers, R. B. (1994) A new concept in maxillary implant surgery: The osteotome technique. Compendium of Continuing Education in Dentistry 15: 152 – 158.

Schwartz-Arad, D. and Samet, N. (1999) Single tooth replacement of missing molars: a retrospective study of 78 implants. J Periodontol 70: 449 – 54.

Tarnow, D., Elian, N., Fletcher, P., Froum, S., Magner, A., Cho, S. C., Salama, M., Salama, H. and Garber, D. A. (2003) Vertical distance from the crest of bone to the height of the interproximal papilla between adjacent implants. J Periodontol 74: 1785 – 8.

Tarnow, D. P., Cho, S. C. and Wallace, S. S. (2000) The effect of inter-implant distance on the height of inter-implant bone crest. J Periodontol 71: 546 – 9.

Tatum, O. H. J. (1986) Maxillary and sinus implant reconstruction. Dent Clin North Am 30: 207 – 218.

Thilander, B., Odman, J., Grondahl, K. and Lekholm, U. (1992) Aspects of osseointegrated implants inserted in growing jaws: A biometric and radiographic study in the young pig. Eur J Orthod 14: 99 – 109.

Westwood, R. M. and Duncan, J. M. (1996) Implants in adolescents: a literature review and case reports. Int J Oral Maxillofac Implants 11: 750 – 5.

Zervas, P. J., Papazoglou, E., Beck, F. M. and Carr, A. B. (1999) Distortion of three-unit implant frameworks during casting, soldering, and simulated porcelain firings. J Prosthodont 8:171 – 9.